Going Green

An Exploit Steeped in Moral Turpitude

Jeff Quinn

"If you're going to say what you want to say, you're going to hear what you don't want to hear."

Alcaeus of Mytilene

Contents

Foreword   7

Part I

History and Use of Cannabis Sativa   15
The Downfall of Hemp   34
Medical Cannabis   50
420   56
Roaches and Culture   62
Rastafarians   66
Quotable   75

Part II

On the Ball   87
Location, Location, Location   95
A Transient Experience   102
By a Camel's Nose...BOS I   106
A Face to face with the Super   115
Lawyers   121
Winter of Our Discontent   124
Fun and Games in Holbrook...BOS II   132

Part III

"You Guys were Mormonized"   145

Tabla Rasa   149

About Schmitt   159

Three's A Charm...BOS III   165

Finger Lickin' Cashew Chicken   169

The Windy Joint   178

Dispirited   182

A Grow Facility Cometh   186

Part IV

Twisting up Loose Ends   191

Altercation at the Compactor   199

The Mutie Chart   205

Same, Same, But Different   209

Postscript   215

Foreword

Who in their right mind wouldn't leap at the opportunity to make a little dinero? Legally of course. Who doesn't desire a new house? A new car? Hell, I'd settle for health insurance. This being said, I came into the marijuana industry kicking and screaming. Well, perhaps not literally, but in any event for several years leading up to my reluctance to 'jump on board' I wanted nothing at all to do with medical marijuana. It wasn't the marijuana aspect of the business that aroused feelings of disinclination. It was a certain fondness for a little blue passport that swayed my thought process. You see, I couldn't and still can't, fathom the thought of being denied access to the world. Money and material objectivity are groovy but certainly not worth – to me anyway – losing the freedom to hop on a plane and discover other cultures. I obviously measure wealth differently than most.

A combination of advancing age and looming economic stagnation (or was it stagflation?) had seriously hampered my opportunities of obtaining gainful (and meaningful) employment. While these factors surely had something to do with my resolution to 'jump on board', the real motivation behind my change in reasoning had to do with my lifelong friend Dusty De Carlo. A medical marijuana dispensary venture in one form or another had been Dusty's dream for as long as I could remember. He'd willingly taken part in so many of my madcap traveling escapades over the years I felt it only right to back his play. So it was, in this interest, of Dusty's dream, that I agreed to embark on the odyssey.

Dusty's dispensary journey began years earlier in a place far, far away – Michigan to be exact – which had then recently passed medical marijuana legislation. Residing in Ohio at the time, Dusty along with our old friend, David 'Guibs' Nardecchia, made forays into southeastern Michigan in search of a town to base their operations. At the zenith of conspiracy, the plot unraveled, Dusty's Michigan field of dreams unraveling along with it. Switching gears, Dusty made tracks back out to Arizona where the issue of medical marijuana was once more under heavy discussion. In November, 2010 the citizen initiative, *Arizona Medical Marijuana Act* (proposition 203), passed by a slim margin. Voters had given blessing to several similar measures over the years but for one reason or another none of these measures ever came to fruition. One must remember we are talking about Arizona here. If there is one thing I've learned in my thirty plus years residing in the state it is this: Never underestimate the zaniness of Arizona politics. Just as you think you've made sense of it all, that you've figured out how the system works, you'll find yourself back at square one, a sense of bewildered wonderment filling your thoughts. If Arizona voters could pass an initiative making Martin Luther King Day a state holiday in order to obtain the Super Bowl, they could surely pass medical marijuana statutes, or so one would suppose.

All signs indicated that the renewed and rejuvenated medical marijuana efforts of 2010 might actually take root and Dusty wanted to be there when and if it happened. In those early days I assisted Dusty by keeping him abreast of the latest news and developments. I ostensibly got the ball rolling by writing an email to a man named Allan Sobel requesting information regarding dispensary licensure and the process it entailed. Dusty, along with his friend Michael, chased down leads and applied for an LLC. They dreamed the dream, impatiently awaiting the day when the state would begin accepting dispensary applications. Just as their excitement peaked the entire process stalled out. Nothing happened for weeks then months. Michael moved to Belize to see if he could make a go at expat retirement. Dusty joined him to see what prospects the country held. In the end they both became disillusioned; returning to Arizona only to discover state officials still hadn't made any progress on the dispensary front. As for me, I journeyed to Taiwan to teach English on the small island of Nangan. Returning nine months later, the dispensary program remained in a holding-pattern. By this time the state had begun allowing doctors to make patient recommendations for medical marijuana cards based on medical criteria such as cancer and chronic pain. The state allowed 'designated caregivers' to supply medical marijuana and 'cultivators' to grow it. Many of these people were one and the same. For instance a patient could also be a caregiver and cultivator. Marijuana was flowing legally but none of it originated or passed through or out of the dispensary system which remained hopelessly inoperable. In this void left by the state's inaction, quasi-legal 'compassion clubs' popped up all over the metro Phoenix area, patients and caregivers exchanging 'medicine' cardholder to cardholder for 'donations' intended to cover their expenses. By its own inaction the state had opened up an unregulated can of worms. Dispensaries were designed to be heavily regulated and bound to statute, compassion clubs on the other hand, were fly by night pseudo-legal entities operating in gray areas. Meanwhile, behind the scenes politicians had their sticky hands on the reins, trying their best to derail the intentions of the voters by undermining the entire medical marijuana program. From the governor and attorney general on down, attempts were made to prevent, or at the very least, delay progress.

Let's face it, marijuana is a polarizing subject. In any democratic society a random slice of the population exhibits strong opinions – both pro and con – stemming from religion and morality to divine right while the majority muddles along feebly in their wake. Just how big is marijuana in the United States? Combining medical and recreational use, the U.S. market ranges somewhere between 15-50 (some experts peg it at around 38 billion) billion dollars. That's bigger than tobacco. Bigger than cotton. A 38 billion industry makes marijuana bigger than wheat and corn combined! Worldwide, some 190 million people use marijuana each and every day. 10% of the population in the United States uses marijuana. A third of those are said to be college students. In 1978, 50% of high-schoolers admitted trying marijuana. Today the number hovers somewhere around 48%. Evidently programs such as *Dare* and *Just Say No* have held little sway.

This book you hold in your hands serves as the record of Overgaard Compassion Care's plight to open up a state legal medical marijuana dispensary in the state of

Arizona. Obviously, I can't speak for other dispensary owners and their own personal triumphs and impediments, as I wasn't involved in their struggle if indeed there was one. For Overgaard Compassion Care it was indeed an uphill struggle of epic proportion. A long and tedious process that took an immense toll on all those directly and indirectly involved. I'd like very much to relay that the celebrations outnumbered the setbacks but by doing so I wouldn't be hoodwinking anyone, most of all myself. It was a long and arduous trek punctuated by bureaucratic folly, serious conceptual misconception, and utter satire.

  In order to set the stage, I decided it was imperative to include pertinent information regarding the background and status of cannabis and the cannabis industry by including both historical data and societal mores concerning the mysterious and often misunderstood *weed* widely known as marijuana.

PART I

Origins

History and Use of Cannabis Sativa

*A*s I sat in my hovel writing this chapter, I began experiencing an eerie feeling of déjà vu. In a previous work on the pawn industry entitled *Pawndemonium*, I had described the arduous undertaking of sifting through reams of nebulous and fuzzy material passing for the history of pawn. Two years later I found myself once more confronted with and confounded by similarly tenuous data as I attempted to sort out fact from fiction surrounding the lengthy history of hemp and cannabis. From what I gather, internet findings are widely accepted as gospel truths. Once something appears on the web it magically becomes *real*, no matter how *unreal* it may sound or appear. As a scrupulous researcher, I try my level best to cross-reference everything I come across until my eyes blush with bleariness and I feel I've satisfactorily exhausted the subject. From what I gather, the timeline of events associated with the industries of both pawn and hemp are rarely challenged or the slightest bit variant simply copied and reproduced *in situ*. Strangely, words from Hitler come to mind: 'The great masses of the people will more easily fall victims to a big lie than to a small one.' I'm not professing here that everything on the internet is incorrect or deceitful; I'm just saying a hell of a lot of it isn't all that well thought out. For instance, when I read (over and over again through cut and paste reposts) that Buddha ate nothing but one hemp seed a day for six years, I thought to myself...Hmmm. Do people find this credible because Buddha is spiritually magical or simply because they read it on a marijuana website so therefore it must be true?

To most living outside the U.S., marijuana is known simply as cannabis, a plant genus comprised of three main categories: *Cannabis Sativa, Cannabis Indica,* and *Cannabis Ruderalis.* Before I get wrapped up in historical conundrum let me take a stab at clarifying the differences between hemp, marijuana, and cannabis. Technically speaking, hemp, cannabis, and marijuana all fall under the scientific Latin denotation *Cannabis Sativa.* According to the feds, hemp refers to the stalks, stems, and sterilized seeds of the cannabis sativa plant while the term marijuana refers to the leaves, flowers, and 'viable' seeds of the cannabis sativa plant. No matter what you call it – hemp, cannabis, or marijuana – it is all illegal under United States federal law. A majority of the marijuana in the world today is a hybrid combination of Sativa and Indica – Indica being a subspecies of Cannabis Sativa. Confused yet? Tetrahydrocannabinol, better known as THC, is the active ingredient found in marijuana; the one that induces a recreational high and supplies relief to medical marijuana patients. Hemp contains very little THC as THC is found mainly in the flowers of the plant. Countries such as Canada authorize hemp production so long as the plant contains no more than .03 percent of THC. The downside of this equation is the fact that very little seeds are produced; seeds with some of the highest nutritional and protein value known to our planet. Hemp is grown in close rows with only a few inches separating each plant. This method produces tall, woody, spindly plants that can reach heights of ten feet or taller. Cannabis grown to produce recreational or medicinal-grade marijuana, on the other hand, is sowed at a distance of 18 inches apart or further allowing the plants to become bushy. This elbow room results in the production of many low, flexible branches. The following is a definition from medical marijuana advocacy group, Americans For Safe Access as stated in their website article *Research: Definitions and Explanations:*

'Cannabis sativa L. is the botanical name and Latin binomial of hemp. Hemp (Cannabis sativa L.) is an annual plant, normally dioecious, with male and female flowers developing on separate plants. Depending on THC and CBD content hemp can be divided into fibre and drug types. There are regional differences in the employment of the terms cannabis, hemp and marijuana. Marijuana (marihuana) is a colloquial name for dried leaves and flowers of drug cannabis varieties rich in THC (1-20% THC). The median content of THC of confiscated marijuana in the USA in 1997 was 4.2%. Marijuana available on prescription in the Netherlands contains 15% or 18% THC. THC (tetrahydrocannabinol) usually refers to the naturally existing isomer of delta-9-THC, but also may include delta-8-THC. Delta-9-tetrahydrocannabinol and delta-1-tetrahydrocannabinol are two names for the same molecule according to different numbering systems (monoterpenoid and dibenzopyran nomenclature). Generally the natural trans-isomer of delta-9-THC of the cannabis plant, the delta-9-trans-tetrahydrocannabinol or dronabinol is designated. Chemically, delta-9-THC is defined as (6aR-trans)-6a,7,8,10a-tetrahy-dro6,6,9-trimethyl-3-pentyl-6H dibenzo [b,d] pyran-1-ol with a molecular weight of 314.47 Da.'

I bet you didn't think you'd ever have to fall back on those high school chemistry classes did you. Here's an acceptable summary of the difference between Indica and sativa by The National Organization for Reform of Marijuana Laws (NORML) posted on their Orange County website entitled *Medical Marijuana Strains*:

'There are really only two sides of the marijuana family we are talking about here. Indicas and Sativas. Sativas are just about the opposite of Indicas. They are tall, thin plants, with much narrower leaves and grow a lighter green in color. They grow very quickly and can reach heights of 20 feet in a single season. They originally come from Colombia, Mexico, Thailand and Southeast Asia. Once flowering has begun, they can take anywhere from 10 to 16 weeks to fully mature. Flavors range from earthy to sweet and fruity. The effects of a Sativa is cerebral, up and energetic. Indicas originally come from the hash producing countries of the world like Afghanistan, Morocco, and Tibet. They are short dense plants, with broad leaves and often grow a darker green. After flowering starts they will be mature in 6 to 8 weeks. The buds will be thick and dense, with flavors and aromas ranging from pungent skunk to sweet and fruity. The smoke from an Indica is generally a body type effect, relaxing and laid back. Indica's higher CBD than THC equals a much heavier, sleepy type of high. Indica plants have a heavy, stony high that is relaxing and can help different medical problems. Combining different Indicas, different Sativas or a combination thereof creates hybrids. The resulting hybrid strains will grow, mature and smoke in relationship to the Indica/Sativa percentages they end up containing.'

~

As I cautioned earlier, one must certainly be wary of the sources professing dates and lineage associated with hemp and cannabis. The history of hemp and cannabis as it pertained to human use (your guess is as good as mine as to how long it had been growing naturally) is very, very old. Just how old? That depends on the evidence or again, lack thereof. Some (I use extreme caution in referring to any of these people as experts) claim hemp was being grown for its fibrous value in Taiwan as far back as 10,000 years ago. Others claim it has been around for over 12,000 years. If this were the case why then does the first relic of woven hemp fabric date back only to around 7000-8000 BCE? I know it's only two thousand years but that's all that separates us today from the time of Jesus and after all, a whole hell of a lot has happened since then.

I read that the Chinese were consuming hemp seeds as far back as 6000 BCE. The first archaeological use of hemp in China dates back to the 5th century BCE during the Neolithic Age when archaeologists discovered hemp fiber imprints on pottery used by the Yangshao culture. China coined the name for hemp in the form of the Chinese character *Ma*. Soon thereafter everything hemp-like from actual hemp to non-hempen jute and ramie were referred to as *Ma, Ta-ma* or *Da-ma* (great hemp).

The Chinese are likewise ballyhooed as being responsible for the first documented use of cannabis for medicinal purposes, said to have occurred around 2727 BCE. Whether seed-munching eased someone's pain in the interval sandwiched between 6000 BCE and 2727 BCE remains uncertain. Here's what I find odd about this so-called 'documentation'. The person responsible for documenting the use is a legend. That's right, a legend. And I don't mean like Larry Bird or Babe Ruth, a legend in the fictitious sense. So if this Shennong is a legend (a la Robin Hood or Lone Ranger) we don't know for certain what, if anything, about the man is real let alone what he may or may not have 'documented'. This sort of factual regurgitation shocks me, but obviously has no bearing whatsoever on those reposting the legend as historically binding. This legendary Chinese 'emperor', 'philosopher', 'inventor', and 'master cultivator' going by the name Shennong, allegedly recommended marijuana for rheumatoid conditions, gout pain, malaria, constipation, 'female pain', and absentmindedness. I don't know about you but that bit about absentmindedness sounds somewhat dubious. I've heard people profess marijuana curing what ails them but I've never heard anyone claim it improved their memory.

Not only was this Shennong responsible for being the first to document his utilization of marijuana but according to legend (there's that word again), he was also the first to discover tea. The story goes that the 'Divine Farmer' (Shennong) insisted that his drinking water be boiled before he drank it so that it would be clean. Makes sense right? He probably bathed once a year but at least he had clean drinking water. One day, on a trip to a 'distant region', Shennong and his army pulled up for a siesta. Was he also a general? As a servant began boiling water for Shennong to drink, a dead leaf from a wild tea bush plummeted into the cooking pot. The tea leaf, turning a brownish color, allegedly went unnoticed before being presented to the parched, multi-talented Shennong. Taking a sip, Shennong found the brew refreshing, and voila...Cha or tea, came into being. Here's my beef with all this. Why would site after site place Shennong on the marijuana timeline if there is any question as to his authenticity? There are plenty of interesting legendary characters scattered throughout history but very few that belong on a historically accurate timeline. Shouldn't it be a prerequisite that a historical timeline contain historically accurate information? Am I missing something here? Here's the bottom line: The legendary Shennong wrote a legendary book about the medicinal prowess of cannabis. End of story. I'll leave the believing or disbelieving entirely up to you. Why not enjoy a cup of tea while you are at it...

From China, hemp's popularity grew steadily, tracing various trade routes southwest into India where it became known as *sacred grass* in Hindu texts such as the *Artharvaveda*. This ancient document describes how the god Shiva brought cannabis down from the Himalayas for his followers' use and enjoyment – both recreationally and spiritually. The following terminology was assigned to the various ways in which Indians utilized cannabis. *Ganja* referred to the flower (bud) and upper leaves of the female plant. *Charas*, often likened to hashish, contained high concentrations of resin and was the most potent of the three preparations. *Bhang,* a cannabis milk beverage, was first used in Hindu rituals around 1000 BC. The spicy beverage, often served at celebrations, included cloves,

21

cinnamon, rosewater and sugar. Though *Bhang* can be used as a general term for marijuana, it is most commonly used only in reference to the beverage. Hemp, still considered one of the five sacred plants of India, has played an integral role in cultural and religious ceremonies as far back as 1500 BCE.

According to the *Sushruta*, a Sanskrit text on surgery, hemp was employed to cure leprosy. Call me a skeptic, but I find this hard to fathom. If the *Sushruta*, written sometime prior to 1000 BCE, got it right then how do we still have over 215,000 people currently living with this monstrous disease? These days the disease is commonly referred to as Hansen's disease, which might sound better, but sure can't feel any better to those afflicted. Historical treatment options included cobra venom, scorpion stings, blood baths…And cannabis.

By 800 BCE, hemp had meandered its way into what is now the Caspian steppe region of modern-day Iran where it is presumed the Scythians gradually spread hemp into Europe and other parts of central Asia. Perhaps best known for the invention of the scythe, the Scythians were given props for their fine hempen garments by the Greek historian Herodotus in 500 BCE. Herodotus described death rituals whereby Scythians, gathering in tents, inhaled vapors from hemp-seed smoke. According to Herodotus, the vapor room thing was done both ceremonially as well as recreationally. For some reason I can't seem to get the image of finely-attired grim reaper-types huddled inside a musty old tent out of my head.

Hemp was cultivated for the first time in jolly old England around 70 AD. By the time 400 AD rolled around hemp had become a well-established English crop, eventually falling under royal decree.

Practicing in Rome under Nero, Greek physician/botanist Pedanius Dioscorides, branded the hemp plant *Cannabis Sativa* while describing its various medicinal uses in his five-volume tome, *De Materia Medica*. Compiled between 50-70 AD and circulated in Latin, Greek, and Arabic, *De Materia Medica* was the precursor of modern pharmacopeia. Dioscorides made note of hemp's particularly strong fibrousness and medicinal properties in *Book III of Materia Medica* stating: 'Kannabis; is a plant of much use in this life for the twisting of very strong ropes, it has leaves like to the Ash, of a bad scent (insect repellent), long stalks, empty, a round seed, which being eaten reduces sexual activity, but being juiced when it is green is good for the pains of the ear.'

Roman author, Gaius Plinius Secundus (also known as Pliny the Elder AD 23-79), discussed the many industrial uses of hemp in his celebrated work, *Naturalis Historia*.

By the year 1000 AD, cannabis as a recreational substance, had become widely popular throughout the Arab world. In a society where alcohol and baby back ribs were strictly prohibited, cannabis (especially in the form of hashish) filled the void. The spread of cannabis use in the Middle East is often attributed to a 14th century mystic named Sayyid Haydar Amuli. Like many a soccer star, the founder of Sufism – which is often described as an esoteric or inner dimension of Islam – was often referred to by the single label Haydar. According to legend (there's that word again), Haydar became depressed and felt the need to leave the monastery compound for a walkabout in some nearby fields. Apparently this Haydar fellow stumbled upon a stand of cannabis plants and made a snack out of the leaves. When he returned to the monastery his followers took note of his relaxed, euphoric state. From that day forward Sufis have enjoyed the relaxing properties of cannabis. Haydar was so enamored by cannabis he requested leaves accompany him in his tomb upon death.

By 1009 AD, hemp-based paper made its way into Europe via the Arabic culture. The first hemp-paper mill in Europe was reportedly constructed in Xàtiva, Spain. Paper production continued under Moorish rule until 1244 when Christo-European armies drove them out. Moors or no Moors, paper was chiefly made from hemp for the next 850 years. In 1215 AD, the Magna Carta was drafted on hemp paper.

Disease and horses weren't the only thing Columbus introduced to the New World. He also brought along Cannabis Sativa with him on his famed 1492 voyage. Incidentally, Columbus's sails and rigging were also made from hemp. In fact from the 5th century onward into the mid-19th century, 90% of the world's sailing ships sported sails manufactured from hemp. Why? Because hempen sails were naturally resistant to salt water. The word canvas is derived from the Greek word for cannabis. The *USS Constitution* ('Old Ironsides') required a whopping 60 tons of hemp for its rigging requirements including a 25-inch (circumference) anchor rope.

By the mid-16th century, European leaders, realizing the importance of hemp, began mandating laws of production. Henry VIII of England passed an act stating that all landowners must sow at least 1/4 acre of hemp or face being fined. In 1564, King Phillip of Spain ordered hemp grown throughout the entire Spanish empire, from present-day Argentina to

24

present-day Oregon. A few centuries later, King George III of England tapped into the spacious fields of North America looking for solutions to remedy hemp deficiencies in Great Britain. While hemp was indeed grown in the colonies, it wasn't the hit King George had counted on, as many farmers gladly paid penalties in the form of taxes for refusing to grow hemp in lieu of growing a more lucrative crop, tobacco.

In 1791 U.S. President George Washington established import taxes on hemp to encourage the domestic industry to flourish. 'Make the most of the hemp seed. Sow it everywhere', rallied Washington. Thomas Jefferson referred to hemp as "a necessity" and urged farmers to grow hemp instead of tobacco. "Hemp is of first necessity to the wealth and prosperity of the nation", pronounced Jefferson. Many get a kick out of the fact that rough drafts of the Declaration of Independence were penned on paper made from hemp. Better yet, one could pay their taxes with the stuff as it was legal tender in America.

As Americans scrambled to stake their claims westward in the 19th century they did so in wagons covered with canvas made from hemp.

The year 1892 ushered in the advent of the diesel engine. Designed by German, Rudolph Diesel, the engine was intended to operate on vegetable and seed oils. While the initial engine unveiled at the 1900 World Fair in Paris ran on peanut oil, Rudolph planned on using a wide array of oils including those obtained from hemp seeds. 'The use of vegetable oils for engine fuels may seem insignificant today, but such oils may become, in the course of time, as important as petroleum and the coal tar products of the present time', said Diesel. Prophetic? Diesel believed the

United States possessed the greatest potential market for his engine. Comprehending the dangers of pollution, Diesel considered his engine a solution to the problems posed by petroleum-based products. In 2011, the United States biodiesel industry produced more than one billion gallons of biodiesel fuel. Are we finally beginning to wake up? The first diesel engine built in the United States was produced in 1898 by Busch-Zulzer Brothers Diesel Engine Company. Adolphus Busch, of Budweiser brewing fame, was the president of the company.

Diesel died under mysterious circumstances in 1913, when he vanished during an overnight crossing of the English Channel en route from Antwerp to Harwich on the mail steamer *Dresden*. Some view Diesel's death as downright fishy while others view it as either accidental or an act of suicide. In any event, Diesel was never seen again after taking dinner and retiring to his room around 10 pm on the evening of September 29, 1913. Before retiring, Diesel had left word to awaken him the following morning at 6:15 am. Diesel never made the wake-up call and furthermore, his bed had not been slept in. Diesel's heavily decomposed body was discovered ten days later near Norway. The only way to identify the corpse as that of Diesel's was by rifling through the contents of the pockets which contained Diesel's wallet, pocket knife, pill case, and eyeglass case. The contents were identified by Diesel's son, Eugen, and the body returned to sea. Conspiracy theorists insist the German government had a hand in Diesel's demise as Diesel had apparently been friendly to France, Britain, and the United States. Shortly after Diesel's death, a diesel-powered German submarine fleet was unveiled. Coincidence?

In 1925, Henry Ford told a New York Times reporter that ethyl alcohol was "the fuel of the future". Ford was merely articulating an opinion that was widely shared at the time in the automotive industry. 'The fuel of the future is going to come from fruit like that sumach (sic) out by the road, or from apples, weeds, sawdust – almost anything. There is fuel in every bit of vegetable matter that can be fermented. There's enough alcohol in one year's yield of an acre of potatoes to drive the machinery necessary to cultivate the fields for a hundred years.' Ford would later produce a car that ran on hemp oil and was constructed out of resin-stiffened hemp fiber.

The term *pot* can be loosely traced back to 1935. The slang word for marijuana stems from the Spanish-Mexican word potiguaya or potaguaya, a shortening of the Spanish-Mexican name for brandy (potación de guaya). Apparently the brandy was steeped with marijuana buds. When translated literally, potación de guaya means *drink of grief*. Somehow that doesn't sound very alluring to me.

In 1937, inaugural Commissioner of the new Federal Bureau of Narcotics (FBN), Harry Anslinger, dealt a crippling blow to the hemp industry by pushing the Marihuana Tax Act of 1937 through congress. I'll discuss the implications and details of the act in the next chapter.

During WW II, a 'Hemp for Victory' campaign was initiated in the United States. Prohibitive taxes levied on farmers as a result of the Marihuana Tax Act of 1937 basically destroyed the hemp industry in the United States leaving it dependent on jute from India and hempen imports from Asia. As Asian countries fell rapidly to Japan the supply chain all but dried up. The

Philippines, for instance, supplied Manila Hemp used to make rope and cordage. However, they were invaded soon after Pearl Harbor was attacked in 1941, extinguishing any hope of acquiring further product. Manila Hemp, named in the honor of the capital of the Philippines, is an interesting misnomer as Manila Hemp isn't hemp at all. Manila Hemp is actually a fiber obtained from abacá (*Musa textilis*), a relative of the banana plant. The name Manila Hemp was assigned as a result of hemp being used for so many years and so many similar fibers were christened as "hemps". Who knows, you most likely have some abacá sitting in your office right now as Manila envelopes and Manila paper are produced from the plant. While nylon and other synthetic fibers have replaced Manila Hemp, India continues to utilize Manila rope to hang convicts. With all the rape cases making the news these days, it appears they'll need a lot of the stuff.

A single WWII era battleship required an incredible 34,000 feet of rope manufactured from hemp. Parachute webbing, boot laces, thread, canvas, textiles, fire hoses – the list goes on and on – were all made from hemp, or hemp-like plants. As the surplus on hand dwindled, the government quickly produced propaganda films such as *Hemp for Victory* offering farmers incentives (subsidies) to grow hemp. Farmers growing hemp were even exempted from military service, as were their sons. "Victory Gardens" of hemp soon popped up in states such as Kentucky, Missouri, and Wisconsin. Hemp cultivation increased by several thousand percent as a result of the campaign.

China is currently the leading producer of hemp followed by much smaller manufacturing efforts in places such as Europe, Chile, and North Korea. Today, the United States imports more hemp than any other country in the world. This sickens me to no end. Even though our farmers here in the United States are hurting, they aren't permitted to grow hemp because the federal government makes no distinction between industrial hemp and cannabis. Over the past decade or so a number of states and nearly a dozen Indian tribes have petitioned to begin growing hemp. Unfortunately, they seem to be waiting in limbo to see what the federal government will do.

Marijuana smokers during the Red Scare of the 1950s were often branded as individuals possessing socialistic and communistic tendencies. This was especially true of counterculture groups such as the Beats (Kerouac and Ginsberg et. al.) and later, the hippies. Then, anyone finding themselves in the disfavor of the government was branded as possessing socialistic and communistic tendencies during the Red Scare.

The Single Convention on Narcotic Drugs of 1961 was an international treaty signed by 161 countries. The Single Convention was in essence the first treaty to prohibit cannabis. The convention also required the phasing out of traditional coca-leaf chewing, which by the way still goes on with great fervor in South American locales. Perhaps betel nut and caffeine should have been included as well...You never know what a pimply-faced teen hopped up on Mountain Dew is wont to do next.

One of the first nations mentioned when discussing marijuana nowadays is The Netherlands, their 'coffee houses' beaming examples of cannabis acceptance. However, it is important to note that marijuana is not legal but rather tolerated in The Netherlands. In an effort to focus on harder drugs such as heroin and cocaine, authorities in cities such as Amsterdam target pushers of hard drugs while allowing coffee shops catering to marijuana users. Recently, Portugal became the first country (of any significance anyway) to pass legislation decriminalizing drug use across the board. Not only marijuana but all drugs. This is something I've always espoused. On the surface it might sound wacky, but the numbers seem to prove that it is not. After decriminalization, crime in Portugal decreased, along with HIV rates and teen usage. Overall use of drugs such as heroin and amphetamines similarly leveled off or dropped. The mystery surrounding drug usage had vanished. Does this mean everyone in Portugal is making sterling choices? Of course not. Shangri La does not exist.

Historical Uses of Cannabis

Like many repressed Americans, I have very little personal experience with hemp-based products. I once heard Willie Nelson boast that hemp can be linked to over 50,000 products. I suppose Willie would know wouldn't he. No matter whether there are 5,000 products or 50,000 products as Willie claims; the point is there are many uses for hemp. Since I don't have the time, energy, or desire to attempt to list all the products associated with hemp, a brief summary of hemp categories will have to suffice. It's important to note that some of the products listed below remain unmanufactured here in America simply because the infrastructure required to produce them is either outmoded or unavailable. Hemp stalks are dried and broken down into two parts, thread-like fibers called the bast and the inside pulp known as the hurd. The bast is spun into thread for textiles and cordage while the hurds are used to make anything from building material to fuel and non-toxic ink.

Textiles and Cordage

As I mentioned earlier, hemp was an integral part of the sailing industry for centuries. At the beginning of the 20th century a combination of steel, the steam locomotive, and Manila Hemp gradually replaced hemp in the manufacturing sector. As far as textile and cordage usages go, an endless variety of products are made from hemp including yarn, twine, rope, carpets, clothing, curtains, upholstery, shoes, backpacks, and towels. Hemp-based fabrics vary in texture and strength from tough, durable materials such as canvas and denim (original Levis were made from hemp) to finer fabrics akin to cotton and silk. Modern clothiers such as famed suit designer Giorgio Armani are currently busy producing hemp clothing. Naturally organic hemp fiber is more absorbent, durable, and insulating than cotton-based fibers. At a rate of 1500 pounds of fiber per acre, hemp easily out-produces cotton which weighs in at 500 pounds of fiber per acre. It is estimated that half of all agricultural chemicals used in the United States are employed in the growing of cotton. Please reread that last sentence.

Building material

Hemp has been used as a building material for centuries. In 600 AD, a bridge made of hemp hurds (mixed with lime) was built in southern France. The petrified bridge remains standing to this day. Modern applications often mirror techniques accomplished through the use of straw-bale architecture.

Fuel

Biofuels, such as those made from corn and recycled cooking grease can easily be produced from the oils found in hemp seeds and stalks. Biodiesel, sometimes referred to as hempoline, can also be produced by fermenting entire hemp plants. While a viable substitute for petroleum-based fuels, I wouldn't look for hemp-based fuels to make large inroads into the market anytime soon as there are cheaper alternatives in the biodiesel market currently available such as raw garbage and weeds (the pesky non-smoking variety). Forms of charcoal, methanol, methane and gasoline, can all be manufactured utilizing hemp hurds. Plant-based fuels such as hemp are known as biomass fuels. Undergoing a distillation process called *pyrolysis*, these biomass fuels burn cleaner and are virtually free from metals and sulfur, meaning they are much kinder than fossil fuels and don't increase levels of carbon dioxide in the atmosphere. Hemp hurds are also used to produce paints, stains, varnishes, lubricants, and sealants.

Food products

To be sure hemp has been a part of human cuisine for centuries. Hemp seeds can be eaten raw, ground into meal, sprouted, made into milk (said to be similar to soy milk), prepared as tea, used as oil, and used in baking. The Italians and Germans utilized hemp for a variety of dishes during medieval times such as soups, pies, tortes, and other delectable dishes. Hemp flour can be used to make anything from cereal and waffles to ice cream and hemp tofu. While I can't say many of those items cause me to salivate, I wouldn't mind trying a bottle or two of Hanfblute Bier, a Swiss hemp beer brewed using hemp flowers. Having never tried any of these fine mouthwatering concoctions, I can't comment on how they may taste. As far as critters are concerned, hemp seed is used to feed birds and bait fish, while hemp core chips are used for animal bedding.

Paper

The inner core of the stalk, or hurd, can be used to produce dioxin-free paper. Hemp-paper is naturally acid-free so it doesn't crack, yellow, or deteriorate like tree-paper products. Hemp-paper can be recycled twice as many times as tree-based paper. Over the span of twenty years, a one-acre hemp crop can produce as much pulp as a 4.1-acre parcel of forestland and uses only a fraction of the chemicals necessary to process tree-generated paper.

Medicine

As this category is basically the crux and justification for our business venture, I'll devote an entire subsequent chapter to its explanation.

The Downfall of Hemp

*H*ow was it that an industrious weed with incredible potential and upside found itself in the crosshairs of American prohibitionists? How did Cannabis become an Illegal substance? Sadly, it was all quite simple. Hemp was a competitor and competitors, like any garden variety pest, must be eradicated at all costs. I have already mentioned some of the many uses attributed to the hemp plant: Paper, fabric, food, fuel, etc., etc. Technological advancements gained during the industrial revolution paved the way for more economical, cost-effective methods of manufacturing. Inventions such as the assembly line meant manufacturers could utilize synthetic fibers and tree-pulp (no one was worrying about deforestation) at a lower cost than hemp. No surprise, many industries began shifting away from hemp as a base product. However, in the early 1930s improvements were made in the techniques employed in the process of producing paper from hemp. Ironically, it was the Department of Agriculture that came up with the scientific break-through. With the utilization of a new machine invented by George Schlichten called a decorticator, hemp stood poised to revolutionize the paper-making industry. Or so one would have thought, as hemp-based paper could be produced at half the cost of its tree-pulp cousin. What once required 300-man hours of work to clear a one-acre field suddenly required only two. Not only had hemp-paper become cheaper to produce but it was also much kinder and gentler on the environment. Hemp, which can grow up to twenty feet in a season, was certainly a more renewable choice than trees, which we all know take years to grow. What's more, hemp didn't require sulfuric acid to process the pulp. Bear in mind however, Al Gore and carbon credits weren't part of the political/environmental landscape of the 1930s.

Getting back to the question at hand, what was the reasoning behind hemp's assassination in the manufacturing industry? While several factors certainly attributed to hemp's downfall one powerfully equipped individual made sure the ball got rolling in the right direction. His name? William Randolph Hearst. His motive? Hearst basically cornered the timber market and saw hemp as a looming threat. As a billionaire media mogul, Hearst had the resources and economic might to prop up or destroy anything and anyone he saw fit. By the 1930s yellow journalism had become a finely-tuned art form. It mattered little if a story was true or not. If told enough times it would eventually stick. Just ask Hitler and Goebbels. Hearst's campaign was so complex that it remains indelibly ingrained in the social fabric even today. The media blitz conducted through Hearst's large network of newspapers, magazines, news reels, and propaganda films left a lasting effect on society. Hearst didn't stop, however, by neutralizing industrial uses of hemp; he targeted recreational cannabis use as well.

Although marijuana had been used recreationally and ceremonially for centuries it didn't hit its stride in the United States until around the 1920s. Perhaps the fact that marijuana gained recreational traction at a time when alcohol was prohibited is no coincidence. After all, alcohol-shunning Muslims had been using marijuana recreationally for centuries. It is also important to note that marijuana shared an equally legal status as tobacco in the United States during the 1920s and early 1930s. Furthermore, it certainly was not considered the evil threat and menace to society it would later become through anti-marijuana campaigns. During Prohibition the government didn't ban corn, sugar, grapes, barley, rye, and other crops associated with alcohol. So, why then did the government ban the hemp plant if it didn't (and still doesn't) get anyone high? Marijuana was routinely prescribed for conditions such as labor pains, rheumatism, and nausea. In fact, doctors continued to prescribe marijuana for at least a decade after it was ostracized in 1937.

Trees weren't the only thing on Hearst's mind when he began to smear cannabis. It was also a way of attacking minorities. A renowned racist, Hearst deplored non-whites of any denomination. By depicting marijuana as a drug used by lowly Mexican peons and crazed black musicians, Hearst knew he could appeal to prejudicial whites in order to sway public opinion against both industrial hemp and recreational marijuana.

Who else stood to lose if hemp trumped trees? A man by the name of Lammont Dupont. Yes, that Dupont. The development of new hemp manufacturing techniques meant the prolific weed could be used to produce fabrics, oils, dyes, and plastics. Dupont, specializing in the chemical variety of these substances, knew he had to prevent hemp from succeeding or risk losing the market share. Dupont also happened to produce tree-pulp paper, and was, at the time, involved in discussions with Hearst to join forces via a multimillion dollar paper arrangement. Throw Dupont's heavy-hitting, millionaire financier, Andrew Mellon, into the mix and you had the makings of a truly powerful anti-hemp lobby.

But wait, there's more. Let's add yet another loop to the chain in the form of someone with administrative clout. Enter Mellon's nephew-in-law, Harry. J. Anslinger. Anslinger had held down the post of Assistant Prohibition Commissioner before being appointed as the first Commissioner of the Federal Bureau of Narcotics (FBN) in 1930. Anslinger worked secretively for two full years before unveiling what would eventually become the Marihuana Act of 1937. Though the act didn't outlaw hemp or marijuana outright, it introduced prohibitive taxes (hemp couldn't be transferred without a tax stamp) which essentially dealt a crippling blow to the hemp industry. While working on the legislation, Anslinger failed to consult experts concerning his grandiose scheme. Fearing opposition, law enforcement officials, farmers, scientists, doctors, and of course, the public, were purposely left out of the equation. During the legislative hearings Anslinger, acting as his own star witness, offered newspaper clippings as evidence to support his pious claims. Only one medical expert, Dr. William Woodward of the American Medical Association, was afforded an opportunity to offer testimony at the hearings. Woodward, disagreeing with much of what Anslinger alleged, pointed out that much of the evidence presented by Anslinger (the newspaper articles etc.) was written and produced by Anslinger himself! Congress, mirroring the vast majority of the American public at the time, had little knowledge of marijuana or hemp and therefore had little to base their opinions. As the hour grew late, a weary congress voted in favor of Anslinger's bill. The matter was obviously deemed trivial as attested by the fact that nobody even bothered to record the vote tallies. Consider for a moment the impact this legislation has had on the American penal system, as prisons are occupied by thousands of people incarcerated for smoking marijuana.

The act received criticism almost immediately, but by then it was too late, things were already in motion. Anslinger, acting as America's first drug czar, took it upon himself, along with J. Edgar Hoover, to rid the United States of cannabis. Remember, at the time, it was politically correct and admirable to ensure that white people continue to use the substances they were supposed to use, namely opium and alcohol. Cocaine was considered a drug used by blacks, while cannabis was used by Mexicans. Prior to penning the Marihuana Act of 1937, which effectively put the kibosh on hemp and marijuana, Anslinger, who described drug addiction as 'murder on the installment plan', preempted the legislation with a campaign of propaganda and racial name-calling to gain support. Here's a glimpse of what Anslinger was preaching at the time:

'Reefer makes darkies think they're as good as white men.' '...the primary reason to outlaw marijuana is its effect on the degenerate races.' '...most are Negroes, Hispanics, Filipinos, and Entertainers. Their Satanic music, jazz, and swing, result from marijuana use. This marijuana causes white women to seek sexual relations with Negroes, entertainers, and any others.'

In fairness to Anslinger and the feds, there were various policies and laws passed by individual states banning marijuana prior to the landmark 1937 bill. From 1930-1935, 24 states outlawed marijuana. If you were to examine a map of participating states, you'd notice that a good chunk of western states were on board with banning marijuana while virtually none of the southern states acquiesced.

Anslinger was a staunch believer that marijuana, like Hansel and Gretel's legendary bread trail, was a prelude to heroin addiction and everything grisly that went along with it. After resigning in 1962, Anslinger's successor's continued to hold this same marijuana to heroin stepping stone belief, a belief by the way, which you still hear tossed around today even though studies have shown (over and over again) that data fails to support such claims. Inexplicably, Anslinger rarely if ever slammed cocaine usage. Anslinger apparently took his skewed views to the grave with him, failing ever to moderate on his stance against marijuana. As late as 1970 he continued to maintain that marijuana led to crazed sexual behavior. Here is what he had to say in an interview with *Playboy Magazine* when asked his opinion on the connection between drugs and sex:

'There isn't any question about marijuana being a sexual stimulant. It has been used throughout the ages for that: in Egypt for instance. From what we have seen, it is an aphrodisiac, and I believe that the use in colleges today has sexual connotations. A classical example of amatory activities is contained in the article 'Hashish Poisoning in England,' from the London Police Journal of July 1934. In this remarkable case, a young man and his girlfriend planted marijuana seeds in their backyard and when the stalks matured, they crushed the flowering tops and smoked one cigarette and then engaged in such erotic activities that the neighbors called the police and they were taken to jail.'

Playboy Magazine, February 1970 (p. 72)

Anslinger's infamous essay, *Marijuana: Assassin of Youth,* originally published in *The American Magazine* volume 124 number 1 (July 1937) offers the reader a first-hand glimpse at the extensive propaganda spread to the masses at the time. For both its historical significance and sheer entertainment value, I decided it was paramount to include snippets of the essay. How you take it is entirely up to you. The tagline on the essay reads:

A weed that grows wild throughout the country is making dope addicts of thousands of young people.

THE sprawled body of a young girl lay crushed on the sidewalk the other day after a plunge from the fifth story of a Chicago apartment house. Everyone called it suicide, but actually it was murder. The killer was a narcotic known to America as marijuana, and to history as hashish. It is a narcotic used in the form of cigarettes, comparatively new to the United States and as dangerous as a coiled rattlesnake. How many murders, suicides, robberies, criminal assaults, holdups, burglaries, and deeds of maniacal insanity it causes each year, especially among the young, can be only conjectured. The sweeping march of its addiction has been so insidious that, in numerous communities, it thrives almost unmolested, largely because of official ignorance of its effects. Here indeed is the unknown quantity among narcotics. No one can predict its effect. No one knows, when he places a marijuana cigarette to his lips, whether he will become a philosopher, a joyous reveler in a musical heaven, a mad insensate, a calm philosopher, or a murderer. That youth has been selected by the peddlers of this poison as an especially fertile field makes it a problem of serious concern to every man and woman in America.

THERE was the young girl, for instance, who leaped to her death. Her story is typical. Some time before, this girl, like others of her age who attend our high schools, had heard the whispering of a secret which has gone the rounds of American youth. It promised a new thrill, the smoking of a type of cigarette which contained a "real kick." According to the whispers, this cigarette could accomplish wonderful reactions and with no harmful aftereffects. So the adventurous girl and a group of her friends gathered in an apartment, thrilled with the idea of doing "something different" in which there was "no harm." Then a friend produced a few cigarettes of the loosely rolled "homemade" type. They were passed from one to another of the young people, each taking a few puffs. The results were weird. Some of the party went into paroxysms of laughter; every remark, no matter how silly, seemed excruciatingly funny. Others of mediocre musical ability became almost expert; the piano dinned constantly. Still others found themselves discussing weighty problems of youth with remarkable clarity. As one youngster expressed it, he "could see through stone walls." The girl danced without fatigue, and the night of unexplainable exhilaration seemed to stretch out as though it were a year long. Time, conscience, or consequences became too trivial for consideration. Other parties followed, in which inhibitions vanished, conventional barriers departed, all at the command of this strange cigarette with its ropy, resinous odor. Finally there came a gathering at a time when the girl was behind in her studies and greatly worried. With every puff of the smoke the feeling of despondency lessened. Everything was going to be all right — at last. The girl was "floating" now, a term given to marijuana intoxication. Suddenly, in the midst of laughter and dancing she thought of her school problems. Instantly they were solved. Without hesitancy she walked to a window and leaped to her death. Thus can marijuana "solve" one's difficulties. The cigarettes may have been sold by a hot tamale vendor or by a street peddler, or in a dance hall or over a lunch counter, or even from sources much nearer to the customer. The police of a Midwestern city recently accused a school janitor of having conspired with four other men, not only to peddle cigarettes to children, but even to furnish apartments where smoking parties might be held. A Chicago mother, watching her daughter die as an indirect result of marijuana addiction, told officers that at least fifty of the girl's young friends were slaves to the narcotic. This means fifty unpredictables. They may cease its use; that is not so difficult as with some narcotics. They may continue addiction until they deteriorate mentally and become insane. Or they may turn to violent forms of crime, to suicide or to murder. Marijuana gives few warnings of what it intends to do to the human brain.

IT was an unprovoked crime some years ago which brought the first realization that the age-old drug had gained a foothold in America. An entire family was murdered by a youthful addict in Florida. When officers arrived at the home they found the youth staggering about in a human, slaughterhouse. With an ax he had killed his father, his mother, two brothers, and a sister. He seemed to be in a daze. "I've had a terrible dream," he said. "People tried to hack off my arms!" "Who were they?" an officer asked. "I don't know. Maybe one was my uncle. They slashed me with knives and I saw blood dripping from an ax." He had no recollection of having committed the multiple crime. The officers knew him ordinarily as a sane, rather quiet young man; now he was pitifully crazed. They sought the reason. The boy said he had been in the habit of smoking something which youthful friends called "muggles," a childish name for marijuana…"

No one can predict what may happen after the smoking of the weed. I am reminded of a Los Angeles case in which a boy of seventeen killed a policeman. They had been great friends. Patrolling his beat, the officer often stopped to talk to the young fellow, to advise him. But one day the boy surged toward the patrolman with a gun in his hand; there was a blaze of yellowish flame, and the officer fell dead. "Why did you kill him?" the youth was asked. "I don't know," he sobbed. "He was good to me. I was high on reefers. Suddenly I decided to shoot him." In a small Ohio town, a few months ago, a fifteen-year-old boy was found wandering the streets, mentally deranged by marijuana. Officers learned that he had obtained the dope at a garage. "Are any other school kids getting cigarettes there?" he was asked. "Sure. I know fifteen or twenty, maybe more. I'm only counting my friends." The garage was raided. Three men were arrested and 18 pounds of marijuana seized. "We'd been figuring on quitting the racket," one of the dopesters told the arresting officer. "These kids had us scared. After we'd gotten 'em on the weed, it looked like easy money for a while. Then they kept wanting more and more of it, and if we didn't have it for 'em, they'd get tough. Along toward the last, we were scared that one of 'em would get high and kill us all. There wasn't any fun in it." Not long ago a fifteen-year-old girl ran away from her home in Muskegon, Mich., to be arrested later in company with five young men in a Detroit marijuana den. A man and his wife ran the place. How many children had smoked there will never be known. There were 60 cigarettes on hand, enough fodder for 60 murders. A newspaper in St. Louis reported after an investigation this year that it had discovered marijuana "dens," all frequented by children of high-school age. The same sort of story came from Missouri, Ohio, Louisiana, Colorado — in fact, from coast to coast. In Birmingham, Ala., a hot-tamale salesman had pushed his cart about town for five years, and for a large part of that time he had been peddling marijuana cigarettes to students of a downtown high school. His stock of the weed, he said, came from Texas and consisted, when he was captured, of enough marijuana to manufacture hundreds of cigarettes. In New Orleans, of 437 persons of varying ages arrested for a wide range of crimes, 125 were addicts. Of 37 murderers, 17 used marijuana, and of 193 convicted thieves, 34 were "on the weed."

ONE of the first places in which marijuana found a ready welcome was in a closely congested section of New York. Among those who first introduced it there were musicians, who had brought the habit northward with the surge of "hot" music demanding players of exceptional ability, especially in improvisation. Along the Mexican border and in seaport cities it had been known for some time that the musician who desired to get the "hottest" effects from his playing often turned to marijuana for aid. One reason was that marijuana has a strangely exhilarating effect upon the musical sensibilities (Indian hemp has long been used as a component of "singing seed" for canary birds). Another reason was that strange quality of marijuana which makes a rubber band out of time, stretching it to unbelievable lengths. The musician who uses "reefers" finds that the musical beat seemingly comes to him quite slowly, thus allowing him to interpolate any number of improvised notes with comparative ease. While under the influence of marijuana, he does not realize that he is tapping the keys, with a furious speed impossible for one in a normal state of mind; marijuana has stretched out the time of the music until a dozen notes may be crowded into the space normally occupied by one. Or, to quote a young musician arrested by Kansas City officers as a "muggles smoker": "Of course I use it — I've got to. I can't play any more without it, and I know a hundred other musicians who are in the same fix. You see, when I'm 'floating,' I own my saxophone. I mean I can do anything with it. The notes seem to dance out of it — no effort at all. I don't have to worry about reading the music — I'm music-crazy. Where do I get the stuff? In almost any low-class dance hall or night spot in the United States." Soon a song was written about the drug. Perhaps you remember:

> *"Have you seen*
> *That funny reefer man?*
> *He says he swam to China;*
> *Any time he takes a notion*
> *He can walk across the ocean."*

It sounded funny. Dancing girls and boys pondered about "reefers" and learned through the whispers of other boys and girls that these cigarettes could make one accomplish the impossible. Sadly enough, they can — in the imagination. The boy who plans a holdup, the youth who seizes a gun and prepares for a murder, the girl who decides suddenly to elope with a boy she did not even know a few hours ago, does so with the confident belief that this is a thoroughly logical action without the slightest possibility of disastrous consequences. Command a person "high" on "mu" or "muggles" or "Mary Jane" to crawl on the floor and bark like a dog, and he will do it without a thought of the idiocy of the action. Everything, no matter how insane, becomes plausible. The underworld calls marijuana "that stuff that makes you able to jump off the tops of skyscrapers."

And, above all, every citizen should keep constantly before him the real picture of the "reefer man" — not some funny fellow who, should he take the notion, could walk across the ocean, but — In Los Angeles, Calif., a youth was walking along a downtown street after inhaling a marijuana cigarette. For many addicts, merely a portion of a "reefer" is enough to induce intoxication. Suddenly, for no reason, he decided that someone had threatened to kill him and that his life at that very moment was in danger. Wildly he looked about him. The only person in sight was an aged bootblack. Drug-crazed nerve centers conjured the innocent old shoe-shiner into a destroying monster. Mad with fright, the addict hurried to his room and got a gun. He killed the old man, and then, later, babbled his grief over what had been wanton, uncontrolled murder. "I thought someone was after me," he said. "That's the only reason I did it. I had never seen the old fellow before. Something just told me to kill him!" That's marijuana!

~

Well? What do you think? Did you laugh hysterically or nod along solemnly? As you catch your breath, let me assure you these thoughts and viewpoints are certainly not as outdated and old-fashioned as you might imagine. Judging by the reception we received at our county meetings, Anslinger's message is to be taken quite seriously. Beware the muggles! A movie of the same title, *Marijuana, Assassin of Youth,* directed by Elmer Clifton hit theaters in 1937. The flick, which included mild nudity for effect (remember, it was 1937 after all), was basically a clone of *Reefer Madness*; a film originally produced in 1936 under the title *Tell Your Children. Reefer Madness* was intended as a church-based propaganda film warning of the dangers inherent to marijuana use. Before being released to the flock, the film was purchased by a man named Dwain Esper, who after a little nip and tuck, released the film onto the exploitation film circuit. With the tagline – 'The Sweet Pill *that* Makes Life Bitter! Women Cry For It – Men Die For It! Drug – Crazed Abandon' – the film became an instant flop. At least until the early 1970s that is, at which time the film gained legendary, albeit comical, acclaim at colleges and universities throughout the United States. I've sat through both films and I still can't decide which one of them is worse.

From 1937 to 1947 the U.S. government spent an incredible 220 million dollars on a campaign to wipe out drugs. Between 1948 and 1963, the government spent 1.5 billion on marijuana eradication alone. From 1964 to 1969 the government spent 9 billion in attempts to exterminate 'the devil weed' scourging the land. To assist its quest, congress passed the Controlled Substances Act of 1970 classifying marijuana right alongside heroin and LSD as a schedule I substance, declaring that:

A.   The drug or other substance has a high potential for abuse.

B.   The drug or other substance has no currently accepted medical use in treatment in the United States.

C.   There is a lack of accepted safety for use of the drug or other substance under medical supervision.

It is important to note that prescriptions may not be written for Schedule I substances. Medical marijuana states such as Arizona skirt the federal edict by issuing "doctor recommendations" so that patients may obtain cards. Without a reclassification there is basically no hope for medical marijuana at the federal level.

The latest attempt to reclassify marijuana was undertaken by Oakland-based, Americans for Safe Access, a marijuana advocacy group. It was the first attempt in the past twenty years. The DEA, blinders tight to their eyes, denied rescheduling, standing by their position that marijuana has 'no known medical uses'. In January 2013, the case went before the U.S. Court of Appeals for the D.C. Circuit but was shot down for lack of scientific evidence that marijuana has any medicinal value. 'The federal government has sought and obtained a patent for the medical use of cannabinoids; yet, it claims in these proceedings that marijuana has no medical use,' – Joseph Elford of Americans for Safe Access in a brief presented to the D.C. Circuit. 'Every independent commission to examine marijuana policy has concluded that its harms have been greatly exaggerated – from the 1944 LaGuardia Report, to President Nixon's 1972 Schaffer Commission report, to the Institute of Medicine's congressionally-mandated 1999 report', said Elford.

What everyone has to understand here is that the DEA has a vested interest in retaining the current classification. Consider the assets it would lose in its feeble War on Drugs – helicopters, manpower, seized vehicles and property including cash. They know marijuana has medicinal value but admitting to it would put them in a rather unpleasant position. So what if ¾ of the American population believes marijuana possesses medicinal value? Who ever said democracy rules?

Medical Cannabis

*A*s I mentioned at the tail end of the opening chapter, medical marijuana is the driving force behind my inclusion in the industry and the very basis for writing this book. Prior to 1937, there were no fewer than 2000 cannabis-based medicines produced by over 280 different companies. Every part of the plant has and is being used to produce medicine: the flowers, seeds, oil, stalk, root, and juices. Cannabis allegedly contains as many as 483 compounds, 85 (some sites list anywhere from 60 to 120) of which are presently at the core of medical and scientific cannabis use. Cannabis is the only plant known to produce cannabinoids, a naturally-produced human compound. Cannabinoids serve as appetite stimulants, antiemetics, antispasmodics, and can also offer certain analgesic effects. The following is a small sampling of the conditions treated by medical-grade cannabis: AIDS/HIV, Alzheimer's, Arthritis, Asthma, Crohn's Disease, Epilepsy and spasms, Glaucoma, Hepatitis C, Nausea, Multiple Sclerosis, Migraine headaches, Tourette's Syndrome, Leukemia, sleep apnea, skin tumors, loss of appetite due to chemotherapy, and chronic pain.

Medical marijuana can be administered or delivered in various ways. Dried buds can be smoked using traditional methods such as hookahs, pipes, bongs, or simply rolled into cigarettes. Through the use of what is called a vaporizer, medical marijuana patients can now obtain medicinal quantities without the harmful by-products associated with burning marijuana in a pipe. Vaporizers boil out active compounds and convert them into gas molecules without actually burning the cannabis.

Medical marijuana can also be delivered into the bloodstream via liquid brews such as teas. For those looking to avoid smoking or vaporizing altogether, capsules or edibles are certainly options. A variety of cannabis-based butters and oils are used to make anything from chocolate chip cookies and brownies to suckers and candy bars. Believe it or not marijuana-inclined chefs are even producing true munchie-type snacks such as popcorn and nachos. On the reality television show, *Weed Wars*, a disabled ex-cop from New York preferred to eat his buds dry. To each his or her own. I once sampled a *Special Happy Pizza* in Cambodia, which was essentially a pizza topped with dry shake. It tasted awful and produced no perceptible effect. Put it this way, it was my first and last experience with Special Happy Pizza.

The sheer number of medical-grade cannabis strains available today is mind-boggling. An endless variety of choices allow patients to select properties best suited to their condition and taste. Get a load of some of the names: Blueberry Kush, New York Diesel, AK-47, Purple Haze, Banana Kush, Blue Dream. Girl Scout Cookies, Chronic, Cotton Candy, Durban Poison, GodCrack, Green Crack, Jack Kevorkian, Jack Frost, Moby Dick, White Widow, Orange Crush, Snow Cap, Spurkle, The Wiz, Killa Crip Kush, THC Bomb, OG Skunk…The list goes on and on.

Indica and Sativa subspecies vary in their medicinal properties and treatments. While effects vary from person to person, Sativa strains tend to produce more of a euphoric high by lifting a person's mood and relieving stress while Indica strains relax muscles and act as general analgesics. Indica also assists with sleep disorders. A cancer patient hoping to relieve the pain from chemotherapy would benefit greatly from the effects of Indica, whereas an individual dealing with depression would receive more benefit from Sativa buds. The active chemicals responsible for the medicinal effects of marijuana are collectively called cannabinoids. Sativa's cannabinoid profile is dominated by high THC levels and low or no CBD (Cannabidiol) levels while Indica's chemical profile shows a more balanced mix, with moderate THC levels and higher levels of CBD. While not inducing an intoxicating high, CBD has proven to work remarkably well in controlling seizures and spasms as well as reducing symptoms of schizophrenia. Scientists have been enthusiastic over recent research regarding CBD's potential to combat cancer-cell growth. Though the full picture is still emerging, studies show CBDs retard cancer-cell growth and control the spread of metastatic breast cancer.

Depending on what a patient requires or desires, he or she can go with a Sativa, an Indica, or a mixture of both. With a host of Indica/Sativa hybrids out there today, a patient can effortlessly select a strain with the right balance for their needs. For instance Blue Dream, a cross of Blueberry and Haze, contains 80% Sativa and 20% Indica. Blue Dream is normally recommended for long-lasting pain relief, nausea, migraines, Bi-Polar syndrome, depression, and anxiety. Killa Crip Kush contains 80% Indica and 20% Sativa. Check out this far-out description from medicalstrains.com's website:

Killa Crip Kush smells like a skunk ejected an ill-smelling fluid when startled. It tastes like juicy fruit having an acid or sharp taste. It is also very high in potency rate. Before attempting to smoke this kind of strain, make sure the refrigerator has plenty of storage for eating and drinking because Killa Crip Kush when too much smoked will make the user crippled or disabled for 2 to 3 hours maximum. It can paralyze the lower trunk and legs if the user's usage is beyond limit. Killa Crip Kush is a hybrid Cannabis plant for being both sativa and indica. This plant can be used as medical Cannabis in either daytime and night time.'

I don't know about you but I tend to avoid anything that might paralyze, cripple, or disable me even if only temporarily. Killa Crip Kush, by the way, is recommended for pain relief and insomnia with warnings that it can be 'hazardous' if used excessively. I guess so. The strains I really find entertaining are those that are meant to be used in the workplace. 'Won't slow you down…' 'You'll remain productive…' Please, does anyone really believe this crap; even the tamest marijuana is going to have some effect on performance.

As of May, 2013 18 states and the District of Columbia have legalized medical marijuana in one form or another. As most are aware, Colorado and Washington voted to legalize recreational use in November 2012 and so far the feds haven't crashed the party. Like most lists, this one will soon become obsolete as states are either added or deleted. The list does however serve the purpose of historical record. Here is a list of active medical marijuana states, year the law was enacted, and legal possession limits:

AK	1998	1 oz. usable; 6 plants (3 mature, 3 immature)
AZ	2010	2.5 oz. usable; 0-12 plants
CA	1996	8 oz. usable; 6 mature or 12 immature plants
CO	2000	2 oz. usable; 6 plants (3 mature, 3 immature)
CT	2012	one-month supply
DC	2010	2 oz. dried; other yet to be determined
DE	2011	6 oz. usable
HI	2000	3 oz. usable; 7 plants (3 mature, 4 immature)
ME	1999	2.5 oz. usable; 6 plants
MA	2012	sixty-day supply
MI	2008	2.5 oz. usable; 12 plants
MT	2004	1 oz. usable; 4 mature plants, 12 seedlings
NV	2000	1 oz. usable; 7 plants (3 mature, 4 imm.)
NH	2013	2 oz. usable
NJ	2010	2 oz. usable
NM	2007	6 oz. usable; 16 plants (4 mature, 12 imm.)
OR	1998	24 oz. usable; 24 plants
RI	2006	2.5 oz. usable; 12 plants
VT	2004	2 oz. usable; 9 plants (2 mature, 7 imm.)
WA	1998	24 oz. usable; 15 plants

For the sake of posterity, let's take a quick glance at some of the arguments on both sides of the medical marijuana debate...

Pro-Side:

Proponents of medical marijuana maintain that marijuana can be a safe and effective treatment for a myriad of symptoms including cancer, AIDS, multiple sclerosis, glaucoma, epilepsy, and nausea. Citing studies from peer-review groups as well as prominent medical organizations, pro-medical marijuana backers insist cannabis is a natural alternative to addictive pharmaceuticals. Proponents like to remind their opposition that marijuana has been used medicinally for centuries, and to date, not one person has overdosed.

Anti-Side:

Opponents argue that medical-grade marijuana is too dangerous to use, lacks the FDA's blessing, and that the availability of legal drugs makes marijuana use unnecessary. People on this side of the fence claim marijuana is addictive and inevitably leads to harder drug use. That marijuana impairs driving ability and leads to impending medical problems. Others contend medical marijuana is merely a front for drug legalization and recreational use.

420

Talk to any medical marijuana patient, or seasoned imbiber of any stripe for that matter, and you're bound to hear a convincing fable behind the meaning of the term 420. Over the years the catchphrase 420 has evolved into a not-so-secretive slogan for all things marijuana related. What was once a furtive line between friends intended to befuddle parents and police officers now graces the front of t-shirts, blogs, websites, and magazines. In other words, there's no 'sliding it by' anyone today. April 20th is widely considered national pot smoking day around the world. Turn on the boob tube that day and you're bound to see throngs of revelers toking up in a park or festival. This year (2013) two people were shot during festivities in Colorado where celebrations honored not only 420 but the recent legalization of recreational marijuana. To bolster attendance, groups offered marijuana tours in 'marijuana-friendly' hotels. Prices started at $500 a pop minus airfare.

So just what is the origin of the term 420? I'll bounce a few theories your way, but bear in mind, these are theories passed down by people spending their afternoons passing around a bong so don't get dismayed when the theories turn out to be a little hazy.

The most popular explanation for the term evolved in the early 1970s at San Rafael High School in California where a group of male students met up each afternoon at 4:20 pm to partake in smoky ritual. They called themselves the Waldos in honor of a favored wall located just off school grounds where they enjoyed hanging out. Apparently they were either playing football or in the band squad, but in any event they all seemed to have had after-school commitments tying them up until the witching hour of 4:20 pm. One version of the story has the Waldos getting wind of a member of the Coast Guard nurturing a secret stash of plants near Point Reyes not far from the Coast Guard station. When things got too risky the Coast Guard member is said to have abandoned ship, leaving his crop untended. Like most tasty rumors tossed around smoke-filled basements, this one quickly gathered steam. Assembling at 4:20, The Waldos initially met at the Louis Pasteur statue outside the school. Troops properly amassed, the boys made haste in a 1966 Impala to the Point Reyes area in search of the mythical free range bud. Along the way they toked up and boasted of their bounty to be. 'We would remind each other in the hallways we were supposed to meet up at 4:20. It originally started out 4:20-Louis and we eventually dropped the Louis,' Waldo Steve told the Huffington Post. The hidden crop proved elusive, as the missions failed to turn up any evidence of the Coast Guard stash. In lieu of this setback, a code word among friends in the form of a jaunty catchphrase for smoking marijuana was born. Parents and teachers hadn't the foggiest as to what the teens were referring to when exchanging the phrase 420. Or so the Waldos surmised.

Another theory suggests a teenager named Brad Bann, known by friends as The Bebe, was the *real* person responsible for coining the term 420. This theory contends that The Bebe, preparing for a bong session on a Saturday afternoon in October 1970, casually looked up at the clock and exclaimed 'it's 4:20, time for bong loads'. After this historic (if that's what you want to call it) bong session, The Bebe was said to have employed the term in all sorts of comical ways, even dragging Abraham Lincoln into the mix by using his famed 'four score and twenty years ago...' phrase. The term apparently spread quickly through The Bebe's network of friends. Oh by the way, The Bebe happened to attend San Rafael High School alongside the Waldos. According to The Bebe, he was the one to coin the term while the Waldos helped to spread it around.

The Waldo's have repeatedly backed up their claims by presenting evidence in the form of an old 420 flag along with letters riddled with 420 references. Of course the Waldo's evidence could also back up The Bebe's claims of the Waldo's spreading the phrase.

No matter who coined the phrase, the intriguing aspect to the story revolves around the fact that the term 420 gradually made its way from a California high school to the vast and hazy pot-smoking world beyond. It has been conjectured (here we go again) that the Grateful Dead might have helped pass things along through their many Deadhead supporters. Apparently, the Dead had grown weary of The Haight Asbury scene in San Francisco which by the late 1960s had become overrun by criminals and con artists. Seeking greener pastures the band and its 'associates' decided to base themselves in the hills of Marin County, where, coincidentally, or perhaps not, San Rafael High School happens to be located. The Waldos crossed paths with

Dead members on a regular basis. A Waldo clan father handled real estate matters for the Dead while an older brother managed Dead sidebands *Too Loose To Truck* and *The Sea Stones*. When interviewed, Bassist Phil Lesh and peacenik/Woodstock emcee/ hippie icon, Hugh Romney, better known to the world as Wavy Gravy, said they weren't quite sure when they remembered first hearing the term but both men thought it could have originated in Marin County. That's well and good but not exactly a huge vote of confidence for the Waldos.

While it seems likely that the term originated (one way or another) in northern California, there are still plenty of people out there touting alternative origins: It honored the day reggae legend Bob Marley died. No. That would be 5-11-81. The numbers mocked the penal code for marijuana in California. No. Not anywhere else either. The number of chemical compounds found in marijuana. Yes, there are an abundance of chemicals found in pot, but...No. Tea time in Amsterdam? No. it's actually 5:30 pm which seems very odd, but then there are plenty of odd things going on in Amsterdam. Not being a tea drinker, I didn't happen upon any tea parties during my stays in Amsterdam but did stumble upon plenty of other oddities. Hitler's birthday? No. Why Hitler's birthday would have anything to do with this is well beyond me. Hitler was no friend to pot smoking or pot smokers. It also happens to be my mother's birthday but I assure you she too had nothing to do with the term 420. The tragic Columbine massacre occurred on April 20, 1999 but there doesn't appear to be a direct correlation between the two. There is some speculation that the massacre was actually planned to be carried out on

April 19 to coincide with the Oklahoma City Bombing and Waco Siege, but a snag in plans delayed it until the following day. The delay led others to speculate that the teen mass-murderers, Dylan Klebold and Eric Harris, might have been Neo-Nazis. We'll probably never know. On a much, much lighter note, I did read that a highway in Ontario, Canada where marijuana was known to grow wild for years, was renamed Highway 420 in 1972. This would mean that word would have traveled fast as the Waldos and The Bebe were just coining the phrase a short time earlier in 1970. Some will tell you that all the clocks in the movie Pulp Fiction were set to 4:20 in every scene. This is a myth. While there were clocks set to that time in the pawn shop scene there were plenty of scenes where the clock portrayed other times. Here's a humorous bit of useless trivia...It still remains a mystery as to how the numerical classification SB420 came to be attached to the 2003 California marijuana bill. It surely had to be done in jest but to my knowledge no one has ever come clean to claim it.

High Times magazine wisely locked up the domain name 420.com in the early 1990s. The magazine then set about spreading the term around by promoting the 420 jingle at various events throughout the world such as World Hemp expos and Cannabis Cup in Amsterdam.

Speaking of befuddlement, I've always found it quite curious as to why people find it necessary to "advertise" their proclivity toward marijuana by wearing apparel festooned with leaves and slogans. Let's see...You're walking around the park in a tie-dyed t-shirt with a huge pot leaf gracing the front of it. Your buddy has long, grungy dreads and a t-shirt sporting a picture of Bob Marley smoking a huge spliff. After getting high behind some bushes near the duck pond you walk back to a car displaying a *Fix the Economy, Legalize Marijuana* bumper sticker. You're absolutely appalled when the police have the gall to single you and your buddy out by pulling your car over for a broken taillight while exiting the park. You're doubly appalled when they ask if you have any marijuana on you. I'm not saying anyone should be rousted by the cops, but honestly, what do people expect will happen?

Let's attack this subject from another angle. I may find advertising marijuana unwise but society as a whole must be somewhat okay with it. Although marijuana is classified on the same level (quite unfairly I might add) with drugs such as cocaine and heroin, I haven't come across many t-shirts flaunting afternoon fixes. Remember those red *Enjoy Cocaine* t-shirts which of course were knockoffs of *Enjoy Coca-Cola*. Guess what, they're still around. A quick internet search uncovered dozens of sites selling them. Okay, so there are cocaine t-shirts and marijuana t-shirts and of course beer and alcohol t-shirts. Just how many ketamine users traipsing around in t-shirts featuring tipsy horses on the front there are out there is uncertain but I'd bet not so many. For all I know there are heroin addicts out there donning t-shirts emblazoned with jaunty images of users stumbling around Zurich's Platzspitz (Needle Park).

Roaches and Culture

Marihuana, a slangy Mexican term for wild tobacco, wended its way across the southern border in the early 20th century as immigrants crossed over into the United States in search of seasonal work and a better life. Over time the letter *h* was swapped for the letter *j* and the rest, as they say, is history. The etymology of the word *marijuana* is rooted in racial slurs directed toward Mexican laborers, who preferred a toke or two at the end of a long day to help them unwind after toiling in the fields all day.

The song *La Cucaracha* is a timeworn Spanish corrida passed down over the years from generation to generation. While exact origins are murky the song is thought to have been around since the 16th or 17th century. It is the Mexicans, however, we have to thank for the song's seemingly boundless lyrical alternatives and societal acceptance. The ballad's popularity soared immensely during the Mexican Revolutionary period (1910-20). I tend to think of the catchy ditty as a children's song but then there are plenty of children's songs out there with underlying meanings such as *Ring around the Rosy* (ties to the Bubonic Plague) and *Pop Goes The Weasel* (insinuations with the pawn industry). While some versions of *La Cucaracha* cater to younger minds others obviously do not. Take for instance the following version, written in both Spanish and English, which contains references to marihuana:

La Cucaracha

Spanish	English
La cucaracha, la cucaracha	The cockroach, the cockroach
ya no puede caminar	can't walk anymore
Porque le falta, porque no tiene	Because it's lacking, because it doesn't have
Marihuana pa' fumar	Marihuana to smoke
Ya murio la cucaracha	The cockroach just died
Ya la llevan a enterrar	Now they take her to be buried
Entre cuatro zopilotes	Among four buzzards
Y un raton de sacristan.	And a mouse as the sexton.

I dug up the following excerpt from American poet extraordinaire, Carl Sandburg:

*When a fellow loves a maiden
And that maiden doesn't love him,
It's the same as when a bald man
Finds a comb upon the highway.*

*The cucaracha, the cucaracha
Doesn't want to travel on*

Because she hasn't
Oh, no, she hasn't
Marihuana for to smoke.

"We are not surprised that in the song of La Cucaracha (The Cockroach), there is a variety of theme. Sunny Spain heard the likes of some of the verses before they married a new tune in Mexico. And for understanding the banter and satire of other stanzas one would require knowledge of the careers of Pancho Villa and Zapata besides an acquaintance with Mexican political and revolutionary history. In 1916 in Chicago I heard the tune and two or three stray verses of La Cucaracha from Wallace Smith and Don Magregor, both of whom as newspaper correspondents with a streak of outlaw in them, had eaten frijoles with Villa and slept under Pancho's poncho, so to speak. Also T.K. Hedrick from down Texas way sang the Cockroach song in Mexican. However, we must not assume that a cockroach is what the Mexican means in singing these verses. It may be a pet name, "The Little Dancer," we are told by Alice Corbin. For F.S. Curtis, Jr., of the Texas Folk Lore Society observes, "A whole dissertation might be written upon the fact that a cucaracha may be either a cockroach or a little, dried-up old maid, and that the term was also used as a nickname for the late Venustiano Carranza; and considerable space might be devoted to explaining that marihuana is a weed, which, when smoked, is capable of producing serious narcotic effects and even causing a homicidal mania." Then he queries significantly, "But of what benefit is such stuff to the songs of New Mexico?" The text here is from

Curtis. He says of the tune, "It strongly suggests a sixteenth century origin, especially with the guitar accompaniment usually used."

[p. 289] *The American Songbag*, Carl Sandburg, 1927

Rastafarians

A book about marijuana would be remiss without the inclusion of the Rasta movement. Nearly everyone has heard of Bob Marley and Peter Tosh of Jamaican reggae fame, but perhaps far fewer know the ins and outs of the movement behind the music and culture which have helped to propel it to the world stage. Contrary to popular belief, marijuana is NOT legal nor has it been decriminalized in Jamaica. Don't let the public image of sidewalk toking fool you into believing you can't be arrested and jailed. It is widely believed ganja, as the Rastas often refer to marijuana, arrived to the island in the possession of indentured servants from India in the 19th century. Many feel marijuana would be legal in Jamaica if it weren't for pressure from the United States to maintain the status quo. Let's have a glance at where this culture of dreadlocks, vegetarianism, and ritualistic ganja use came from.

While the official Rastafari movement is generally considered to have commenced with the crowning of Haile Selassie I in 1930, the movement had taken root in the Jamaican slums under the tutelage of Jamaican, Marcus Garvey, in the 1920s. Garvey led an assertive 'Back to Africa' campaign preaching under the pretext that Africans are the true Israelites, having been exiled to Jamaica and other parts of the world as divine punishment. His message, like most messages of change, appealed primarily to the oppressed classes dwelling in the slums where they lived in dire poverty and inequality. Garvey, often regarded by Rastas as a second coming of John the Baptist, peddled a message of black pride while working diligently to reverse centuries of deep-seated feelings tied to enslavement and disentitlement. In 1927, Garvey famously prophesized: 'Look to Africa, for there a king shall be crowned.'

In the eyes of true believers, Garvey's rousing prophesy rang spot-on when Haile Selassie I, Emperor of Ethiopa (1930-1974), was crowned on November 2, 1930. The emperor's birth name, Ras Tafari Makonnen, is where the movement's name is derived. Selassie, at the heart of the Rasta movement, is worshiped as a Jesus incarnate – a messiah. To Rastafarians, Selassie's timely coronation was vivid evidence of Revelation 5:5, Ezekiel 28:25. Haile Selassie means *Might of the Trinity*. The ruler also went by the titles *Conquering Lion of the Tribe of Judah*, *Elect of God*, and *King of the Kings of Ethiopia*. The titles, traditionally bestowed upon Ethiopian kings, reflect an Old Testament emphasis on Ethiopian Christianity. As students of Garvey's teachings, Rastafarians were taught to believe the period of divine punishment had concluded and a return to Africa had begun. Selassie was perceived, at least by Rastas, as the physical presence of God (known as *Jah*) on earth.

As Jamaicans busied themselves hailing Selassie, the Ethiopian Orthodox Christian emperor, seeking to distance himself from the clamor, denied having any divine status at all. In a radio interview with Canada's CBC news in 1967, he explained, 'I have heard of that idea [that I am divine]. I also met certain Rastafarians. I told them clearly that I am a man, that I am mortal, and that I will be replaced by the oncoming generation, and that they should never make a mistake in assuming or pretending that a human being is emanated from a deity.' Obviously Selassie's repudiations failed to deter Rastafarians from believing he was divine. Perhaps they believed he was just being modest. That or he was deliberately trying to remain an emperor on the down low.

Interestingly, for all of Garvey's premonitions and prophesizing, he didn't see eye to eye with the man 'destined' to change the world. Garvey considered Selassie an incompetent leader under the spell of white oppressors such as the meddling British who assisted him to regain his throne in 1944. Ethiopia's independence was put on hold during the Italian occupation lasting formally from 1936–1941 and informally in the form of an Italian guerilla campaign right up through 1943.

As for Selassie's contributions to his country, he worked to modernize Ethiopia by launching the nation into the mainstream of African politics. Bringing Ethiopia into the League of Nations and the United Nations, Selassie decreed the city of Addis Ababa to be the major center for the Organization of African Unity. Selassie's accolades included being named *Time* magazine's Person of the Year for 1935. Selassie was the first black person to appear on the cover in 1930 and the only black leader recognized by the rulers of Europe. These accolades obviously didn't sit well with Garvey who was looking to break free completely from what he viewed as the wicked 'whiteness' of the world.

Haile Selassie first met with Rasta elders in Addis Ababa in the 1950s. In 1955, he offered 500 acres of his personal land to blacks wishing to return to Africa.

Around 2,200 people, mainly Rastafarians, took Selassie up on the offer and moved to the designated land during the 1960s. Unfortunately, the experiment wasn't all that it was cracked up to be. Native Ethiopians cared little about Selassie's Rastafarians and their plans for African rebirth. Moreover, Rastafarians didn't have to travel all the way to East Africa to live in poverty; they could have stayed in Jamaica for that. Today, the Rastafarian population in Ethiopia hovers at around 250. So much for rebirth. While researching I often wondered if there were any white Jamaicans interested in converting to Rastafari and if so would they be referred to as Wastafari?

In 1966, Selassie made an appearance in Jamaica. True believers took it as a sign from God when a severe drought plaguing the island ended abruptly upon Selassie's arrival. As for Selassie, his message went along the lines of warning Rastafarians to stay in Jamaica until they could liberate the island. The slogan *Liberation before Repatriation* echoed throughout Rasta circles. Just how and when this was going to happen remains unclear. Bob Marley's wife, Rita, allegedly converted to the Rastafarian religion after first laying eyes on Selassie, instantly convinced of his divinity. The day of Selassie's arrival, April 21, is celebrated as a Rastafarian holiday.

Selassie was overthrown by means of a military coup in 1974 and kept under house arrest until he was apparently killed by his captors in 1975. Many Rastas held that his death was nothing more than a cruel hoax, that he lives on in hiding until the Day of Judgment. Others maintain that he lives on through individual Rastafarians. Perhaps he plays dominoes with Elvis?

The Jamaican Rasta movement picked up steam in the 1930s as changes began occurring in the slums. With these changes came distinctive hairstyles (the dreads), music, art, and of course lilting lingo. Leonard Howell emerged as an early leader of the movement teaching what he called the six fundamental Rastafarian principles: 1. Hatred for the White race. 2. The complete superiority of the Black race. 3. Revenge on Whites for their wickedness. 4. The negation, persecution, and humiliation of the government and legal bodies of Jamaica. 5. Preparation to go back to Africa. 6. The acknowledgement of Emperor Haile Selassie as the Supreme Being and only ruler of Black people. It isn't difficult to imagine why most of Howell's principles bit the dust and were abandoned as the Rastafarian movement developed and matured. It's often hard to push peaceful agendas when you preach hatred and revenge. Howell was arrested by the Jamaican government in 1933 for demonstrating a loyalty to Selassie in lieu of English King, George V. Howell's arrest could certainly have contributed to the movement's future decision to remain leaderless and independent.

There are currently around one million adherents worldwide. It's important to note many Rastas refrain from using the term *Rastafarianism* saying the *ism* portion of the moniker characterizes an oppressive and corrupt white society. Rastafari is often viewed as a movement as opposed to an actual religion.

As I mentioned earlier, Rastafarians believe in the Judeo-Christian God, whom they refer to as *Jah*. With an emphasis on Old Testament laws, Rastafarian beliefs are rooted in Judeo-Christian dogma and the prophecies foretold in the Book of Revelation. Similar to Christianity, Jah was represented on earth by Jesus (although a darker version) and through Haile Selassie, to whom they refer to as His Imperial Majesty or H.I.M. (pronounced *him*). As I mentioned earlier Rastafaris refer to Selassie as if he were still alive, treating his death as a hoax. Rastafarians also honor Old Testament prophets such as Moses and Elijah. The real differences between Rasta views on Christianity and let's say a Catholic or Protestant view lie in the fact that they do not believe in an afterlife, instead considering Africa (their Zion) as a heaven on earth. I suppose it depends on where in Africa they are placing there gaze. Rastas, at least the true believers, are considered to be physically and spiritually immortal, a concept they call *everliving*. Rastafarians refrain from using the phrase 'you and I', replacing it instead with 'I and I' in order to emphasize the direct line between God and humanity, as well as equality between humans. The division between blacks and whites is a running theme to Rastafarians. The construct, which they call *Babylon*, refers to a historically white power structure maintained by Europeans and Americans to keep blacks in their place by preserving a state of poverty, illiteracy, and inequality. Rastas seek to resist Babylon at all costs countermanding greed and exploitation by acting modest a return to nature as evidenced by their diet.

The *Holy Piby* (Black Man's Bible, not to be confused with the Ebonics Bible) is considered the sacred text of the Rastafari movement. Compiled by Robert Athlyi Rogers of Anguilla from 1913 to 1917, the text was first published in 1924. The *Holy Piby* is basically a version of the Christian Bible which has been altered to remove all the deliberate distortions that are believed to have been made by white leaders during its translation into English.

Modern Rastafari consists of three main sects or orders. Each sect upholds the divine status of Haile Selassie and the importance of black images of divinity; however, the majority of Rastafari do not *belong* to any one sect, choosing instead to maintain a loosely defined organizational makeup. *The Nyahbinghi Order*, named for Queen Nyahbinghi of Uganda, who fought against colonialists in the 19th century, is the oldest of the orders, focusing chiefly on Haile Selassie, Ethiopia, and the eventual return to Africa.

Bobo Shanti was founded by Prince Emanuel Charles Edwards in Jamaica in the 1950s. *Bobo* means black and *Shanti* refers to the Ashanti tribe in Ghana, from which this sect believes Jamaican slaves are descended. Members of Bobo Shanti are alternately known as Bobo Dreads. Donning long flowing robes and turbans over their dreads, the Bobo Shanti observe Jewish traditions and law, including the observance of the Sabbath from sundown Friday to sundown Saturday. The Bobo Shanti differs from the Nyahbinghi in that they worship Prince Emanuel (in addition to Haile Selassie) as a reincarnation of Christ and an embodiment of Jah (God). Emphasizing an eventual return to Africa and reparations for enslavement, the Bobo Shanti chooses to live separately from other Rastafarians, growing their own produce and making money by selling straw hats and brooms. The Bobo Shanti are often seen carrying brooms around with them to symbolize their cleanliness.

The last sect of the trio, the *Twelve Tribes of Israel*, was founded in 1968 by Dr. Vernon "Prophet Gad" Carrington. This is the most liberal of the three

Rastafarian orders and members are free to worship in a church of their choosing. Each member of the sect belongs to one of the 12 Tribes (or Houses), determined by birth month and represented by a certain color.

Since this is after all a book about marijuana, let's take a look at how the plant is used within the movement. Rastas refer to marijuana as ganja (from the Sanskrit word *ganjika*), the holy herb, iley, callie, kaya or other such names. The plant grows abundantly in Jamaica and is believed by Rastas to be a gift from God to be used as a holy sacrament especially when insight from Jah is necessary. To a Rasta, cannabis is a cleansing agent for the body and mind, its properties bringing them nearer to Jah while offering pleasure and peace. Marijuana as a religious article is used primarily during the two main Rastafari rituals known as *reasonings* and *nyabingi*. The *Reasoning* is a casual, informal gathering, in which small groups of Rastas smoke ganja and engage in discussion. I know what you're thinking, this sounds like a party. The ritual begins when one person lights the *chalice*, or pipe then proceeds to recite a short prayer while all other partakers bow their heads. The pipe is passed around the circle until all of the people have imbibed. The ceremony concludes after each participant has departed one at a time.

Nyabinghi, or *binghi* for short, is a dance held during Rasta holidays and special occasions such as Selassie's coronation (November 2) or Marcus Garvey's birthday (August 17). The dances, marathon affairs lasting as long as several days, attract Rastafarians from all over Jamaica. Camping in tents, the formal dances take place at night with reasoning and rest taking place during the day. These dances can last for several days and bring

73

together hundreds of Rastafarians from all over Jamaica. In addition to ritualistic use of marijuana, Rastafarians also use cannabis medicinally for a variety of ailments.

Aside from the use of ganja, perhaps the most telling practice held by Rastafarians is the iconic hairstyle. Dreadlocks serve multiple purposes to a Rasta. The long tresses represent strength in the form of the Lion of Judah (Selassie) and his mane. Since dreads go uncut, they also adhere to the biblical command in Leviticus 21:5 to refrain from cutting one's hair.

The colors red, gold, and green all carry significance to Rastafarians. Red symbolizes the triumphant church and the blood of martyrs in their struggle for liberation. Gold embodies the wealth of the African homeland while green represents Ethiopia's lush vegetation and splendor.

Orthodox Rastas, if such a term exists, obey dietary laws called *Ital*. Under Ital, processed foods are avoided at all costs. Natural foods (eaten as raw as possible) as opposed to canned or chemically-preserved are part of the diet. For this reason most Rastafarians are vegetarian, which makes sense, as it would be easier to adhere to the diet that way. Coffee and milk are also rejected as unnatural. I'd understand this better if they said Coca Cola, but it seems to me that coffee and milk can be consumed naturally if one wished. Rastas also eschew pork and shellfish, paying heed to the Old Testament. Alcohol is also rejected. Due to the process of fermentation, alcohol is deemed unnatural and therefore does not belong in the body. Marijuana, being natural is on the worthy list. Like upright Muslims, alcohol bad, ganja good...

Quotable

*H*ere are a few hand-picked quotes from various individuals pertaining to marijuana and hemp:

"The prestige of government has undoubtedly been lowered considerably by the prohibition law. For nothing is more destructive of respect for the government and the law of the land than passing laws which cannot be enforced. It is an open secret that the dangerous increase of crime in this country is closely connected with this."

–Albert Einstein

"Why use up the forests which were centuries in the making and the mines which required ages to lay down, if we can get the equivalent of forest and mineral products in the annual growth of the hemp fields?"

–Henry Ford

"I think people need to be educated to the fact that marijuana is not a drug. Marijuana is an herb and a flower. God put it here. If He put it here and He wants it to grow, what gives the government the right to say that God is wrong?"

–Willie Nelson

"Even if one takes every reefer madness allegation of the prohibitionists at face value, marijuana prohibition has done far more harm to far more people than marijuana ever could."

–William F. Buckley Jr.

"Casual drug users should be shot."

–Daryl Gates, former Los Angeles Police Chief

"One's condition on marijuana is always existential. One can feel the importance of each moment and how it is changing one. One feels one's being, one becomes aware of the enormous apparatus of nothingness -- the hum of a hi-fi set, the emptiness of a pointless interruption, one becomes aware of the war between each of us, how the nothingness in each of us seeks to attack the being of others, how our being in turn is attacked by the nothingness in others"

–Norman Mailer

"When a private enterprise fails, it is closed down; when a government enterprise fails, it is expanded. Isn't that exactly what's been happening with drugs?"

–Milton Friedman

"It really puzzles me to see marijuana connected with narcotics...dope and all that crap. It's a thousand times better than whiskey – it's an assistant – a friend."

–Louis Armstrong

"That is not a drug. It's a leaf."

–Arnold Schwarzenegger

"I now have absolute proof that smoking even one marijuana cigarette is equal in brain damage to being on Bikini Island during an H-bomb blast."

–Ronald Reagan

"When I was a kid I inhaled frequently. That was the point."

–Barack Obama

"When I was in England, I experimented with marijuana a time or two, and I didn't like it, and I didn't inhale, and I never tried again."

–Bill Clinton

"I think pot should be legal. I don't smoke it, but I like the smell of it."

–Andy Warhol

"The illegality of cannabis is outrageous, an impediment to full utilization of a drug which helps produce the serenity and insight, sensitivity and fellowship so desperately needed in this increasingly mad and dangerous world."

–Carl Sagan

"If John Lennon is deported, I'm leaving too...with my musicians…and my marijuana."

–Art Garfunkel

"We shall, by and by, want a world of hemp more for our own consumption."

–John Adams

"Penalties against possession of a drug should not be more damaging to an individual than the use of the drug itself; and where they are, they should be changed. Nowhere is this more clear than in the laws against possession of marihuana in private for personal use... Therefore, I support legislation amending Federal law to eliminate all Federal criminal penalties for the possession of up to one ounce of marihuana."

–Jimmy Carter

"I enjoy smoking cannabis and see no harm in it."

–Jennifer Aniston

"I would absolutely never use the federal government to enforce the law of using marijuana"

–Ron Paul

"You bet I did and I enjoyed it." (On whether he has ever smoked marijuana)

–Michael Bloomberg

"I think that marijuana should not only be legal, I think it should be a cottage industry. It would be wonderful for the state of Maine. There's some pretty good homegrown dope. I'm sure it would be even better if you could grow it with fertilizers and have greenhouses."

–Stephen King

"When even one American who has done nothing wrong is forced by fear to shut his mind and close his mouth, then all Americans are in peril."

–Harry S. Truman

"Our youth can not understand why society chooses to criminalize a behavior with so little visible ill effect or adverse social impact... These young people have jumped the fence and found no cliff. And the disrespect for the possession laws fosters a disrespect for laws and the system in general... On top of this is the distinct impression among the youth that some police may use the marihuana laws to arrest people they don't like for other reasons, whether it be their politics, their hair style or their ethnic background." "Federal and state laws (should) be changed to no longer make it a crime to possess marijuana for private use." ; "State laws should make the public use of marijuana a criminal offense punishable by a $100 fine. Under federal law, marijuana smoked in public would merely be subject to seizure."

–Richard M. Nixon

"If people let government decide which foods they eat and medicines they take, their bodies will soon be in as sorry a state as are the souls of those who live under tyranny."

–Thomas Jefferson

"We did not view marijuana as a significant health problem--as it was not....Nobody dies from marijuana. marijuana smoking, in fact, if one wants to be honest, is a source of pleasure and amusement to countless millions of people in America, and it continues to be that way."

–Peter Bourne, President Jimmy Carter's Drug Czar in a 2000 PBS Frontline interview

"I support decriminalisation. People are smoking pot anyway and to make them into criminals is wrong. It's when you're in jail you really become a criminal."

–Paul McCartney

"Marijuana is the finest anti-nausea medication known to science, and our leaders have lied about this consistently. [Arresting people for] medical marijuana is the most hideous example of government interference in the private lives of individuals. It's an outrage within an outrage within an outrage."

–Peter McWilliams, American self-help author
"I'd like to see the government back a programme of research into the medical properties of cannabis and I do not object to its responsible use as a recreational relaxant."

–Richard Branson

"Marijuana is self-punishing. It makes you acutely sensitive, and in this world, what worse punishment could there be?"

–P.J. O'Rourke

"Researchers have discovered that chocolate produces some of the same reactions in the brain as marijuana. The researchers also discovered other similarities between the two but can't remember what they are."

–Matt Lauer

"Marijuana is like Coors beer. If you could buy the damn stuff at a Georgia filling station, you'd decide you wouldn't want it."

–Billy Carter

"Smoking's a way to let you down slowly from a ballgame. It also makes you use less of the resources around. It makes people better in the way they act towards society. Everybody's nicer. It's hard to be mean when you're stoned."

–Spaceman Bill Lee, former major league pitcher

"Marijuana is a much bigger part of the American addiction problem than most people - teens or adults - realize."

–John Walters, Former Drug Czar

"The drug is really quite a remarkably safe one for humans, although it is really quite a dangerous one for mice and they should not use it."

–J.W.D Henderson, Director of the Bureau of Human Drugs, Health and Welfare, Canada

"If the words "life, liberty and the pursuit of happiness" don't include the right to experiment with your own consciousness, then the Declaration of Independence isn't worth the hemp it was written on."

–Terence McKenna, American philosopher, writer, lecturer

"Whenever the people are for gay marriage or medical marijuana or assisted suicide, suddenly the "will of the people" goes out the window."

–Bill Maher

"Herb is the healing of a nation, alcohol is the destruction."

–Bob Marley

"In strict medical terms marijuana is far safer than many foods we commonly consume. For example, eating 10 raw potatoes can result in a toxic response. By comparison, it is physically impossible to eat enough marijuana to induce death. Marijuana in its natural form is one of the safest therapeutically active substances known to man. By any measure of rational analysis marijuana can be safely used within the supervised routine of medical care."

–Francis Young, former DEA Administrative law judge

"The drug war is a total scam, prescription drugs kill 300K a year, while marijuana kills no one, but they spend billions/year 'fighting' it, because pot heads make for good little slaves to put into private prisons, owned by the banks who launder the drug money, and it's ALL DOCUMENTED."

–Alex Jones

"Forty million Americans smoked marijuana; the only ones who didn't like it were Judge Ginsberg, Clarence Thomas and Bill Clinton."

–Jay Leno

"If organized religion is the opium of the masses, then disorganized religion is the marijuana of the lunatic fringe."

–Kerry Thornley, co-founder of Discordianism

"Congress should definitely consider decriminalizing possession of marijuana... We should concentrate on prosecuting the rapists and burglars who are a menace to society."

– Dan Qualye

"Some of my finest hours have been spent on my back veranda, smoking hemp and observing as far as my eye can see."

–Thomas Jefferson

PART II

The Plight of Overgaard Compassion Care

On the Ball

*A*s I alluded to in the foreword, I wasn't officially involved with the business at the onset. Technically speaking anyway. I *was involved* to the extent I assisted Dusty in any way I could by researching laws or by writing emails, correspondence, and letters of introduction whenever the need arose. The citizen-initiated Arizona Medical Marijuana Act known as Proposition 203 passed by a razor-thin margin in the November, 2010 election. To give you an idea of the tenuousness of the issue, the measure passed by a positive count in only three Arizona counties (Coconino, Santa Cruz, and Pima). Like most bureaucratic undertakings, progress on the act moved at a snail's pace. It wasn't until April, 2011 that the state finally began issuing identification cards to qualifying patients. The problem was there were no dispensaries set up to supply the cardholders with medical-grade (or any grade for that manner) marijuana. To remedy this glaring glitch in the system, patients were given the right to grow 12 plants for themselves as long as they applied for a cultivator's card. Furthermore, a patient could also apply to be a caregiver for up to five patients besides themselves. This basically meant a patient/caregiver supporting five patients had the potential to grow up to 72 plants in their home. Medical marijuana soon began flowing throughout the state from one cardholder to another as transactions of up to 2 ½ ounces were deemed kosher. As for dispensaries, the state had yet to hammer out the details. The vacuum created by the state's delay opened a gaping maw for pseudo-dispensaries known as 'compassion clubs'. Unofficial and unregulated, these entities operate under the radar by encouraging and conducting cardholder to cardholder transactions. Some compassion clubs act as chummy neighborhood clubs whereby members pay a fee allowing them to hang out and smoke marijuana. Other entities call themselves 'consultation centers' whereby patients receive 'consultations' before donating a prearranged sum for medical marijuana. The consultation/donation fee is intended to cover tangible expenses incurred by the grower such as water, electricity, soil additives etc. Recovering labor costs involved with growing the marijuana is prohibited. However, there are no set guidelines for the 'donation fees' and this ambiguity immediately began causing problems as some patients assumed they should donate a buck or two for a hundred dollars' worth of medical-grade marijuana. Several patients actually called the police complaining that they had been fleeced. The complaints, however, haven't seemed to dampen the climate as plenty of these establishments remain open. So many of these places cropped up that people often confuse them for official dispensaries, a trend that continues even now. Along with the boom came raids and arrests from authorities. If the state had only planned more thoughtfully, the circus-like atmosphere surrounding compassion clubs could have been completely avoided. You know what they say about hindsight...

As I mentioned, the law allows cardholder to cardholder transactions of up to 2 ½ ounces. No paperwork is required. With marijuana 'legally' flowing here, there, and everywhere I suppose it was inevitable that cardholding patients would begin advertising on sites such as Craigslist. Simply place your ad along with a few tasty pics and off you go. In theory the ruse is bulletproof. Barring being beaten and robbed at the point of sale, a cultivating cardholder stands to make a substantial amount of money. Unfortunately, in this age of technology it is often difficult to be sure the person on the other end of the transaction is legitimate. By legitimate I'm referring to a person possessing a valid card? Better yet, is the person on the other end of the transaction an undercover police officer checking to make sure everything is on the up and up? Though the advertising rates are certainly palatable, I'm not sure the risk is warranted. Case in point, earlier this summer an Arizona medical marijuana patient in Phoenix boldly advertised his wares on Craigslist. The man's first undoing was advertising prices at which his various strains were going for. By doing so he was technically breaking the law. According to statute, cardholder to cardholder transactions must be completed strictly on a 'donation' basis. Everyone, including the cops, view the whole 'donation' thing as a sham. Who in their right mind is going to go through all the trouble and expense of growing high-quality medicinal-grade marijuana just to give it away for a few bucks? Had the man run the ad without prices he might have been alright but this too is debatable.

The second miscue occurred when the cardholding Craigslist advertising patient/dealer met an undercover police officer in a Walgreens parking lot. Had he not advertised his prices on Craigslist and had he more carefully handled the future transaction – which reportedly took place by text message – he might have been safe. The advertisement of prices on Craigslist, however, allowed the police to pull him over soon after completing the transaction.

The man's third blunder occurred when he was pulled over down the road from the Walgreens parking lot with a pound plus of marijuana and a bag of meth in his backpack. What started out as a 'can't miss opportunity' wound up going horribly wrong. Here's my question...Is this really worthy of police time? Wouldn't their time be better served chasing down high-level cartels and 'mules' transporting marijuana over the border?

~

In early 2012, Arizona Department of Health Services (ADHS) announced they would begin accepting dispensary applications beginning in May. After some soul-searching, I signed on to the project along with Dusty and Bob 'Bobby' Fern, a retired professor/civil servant in his early sixties. Putting our heads together the three of us painstakingly began poring over the lengthy application required by the state. In addition to a colossal checklist and business plan, the state also required an applicant to show documentation that they possessed $150,000. Lacking funding, we found a patron saint willing to back the project by parking funds for as long as necessary. As for the business plan...We faked it. What I mean to say is we created one by purchasing a ready-made business plan off the internet. After entertaining offers by several people to the tune of $2,500, I concluded I could adapt a generic $14.99 version to meet our needs. Stuffing the template graphs and pie charts with rhubarb and carrots, I managed to somehow make the plan sound convincing.

I think I did anyway. For all I know the state never bothered to read it. With the business plan complete and the application checklist crossed-off, we mailed the whole enchilada to the state along with a check for $5,000. Although they initially said the $5,000 application fee was non-refundable, they ultimately decided to refund a paltry $1,000 back to those who were unsuccessful in obtaining the license.

Soon after handing in the application, Dusty's sister, Heather DeCarlo, placed her cards on the table by agreeing to enter the venture. Bob and I were basically incognito on the paperwork meaning if Dusty had an untimely run-in with a city bus or bolt of lightning the business perished along with him as dispensary licenses, unlike liquor licenses, are non-transferrable.

After all the long hours and hard work was completed all we could do was sit back and wait for a decision from the state. At the application deadline in May it was still very uncertain how the state would go about selecting winners from each CHAA or Community Health Analysis Area. If the state was uncertain, you better believe we all were. Rumor had it the state was going to approve licensure based on the merits of an applicant's business plan and overall application. We also heard an applicant's bank account could sway a decision. Adapted from historical cancer study areas, 126 CHAAS were originally up for grabs. The idea was that for every ten pharmacies one dispensary would be allocated. Tossing federally-administered Indian reservations out of the mix due to the anti-marijuana stance taken by the feds the number of eligible CHAAS was reduced from 126 to 99. Some CHAAS had as many as 14 applicants vying for a single license. I wondered how the state could possibly narrow down the field if every applicant had completed the application correctly. In our CHAA there were only two applicants – a fifty-fifty chance. Despite all the hoopla concerning administrative and substantive review of applications as part of a two-step process, in the end, it was determined each applicant's fate would ride on the whims of a floating ping pong ball. After all the breezy rhetoric, the state decided it was simply too problematic to distinguish between applications, electing instead to employ an air-driven lottery machine to pick winners from each designated CHAA. So much for $2,500 business plans...

Winning the Lottery...

Unless you're referring to the 1948 short story, The *Lottery*, written by Shirley Jackson, I'm not a big fan of lotteries, viewing the practice as yet another way of bilking the poor out of money they don't have. A recent national Powerball jackpot worth over $500 million sold oodles of tickets. A staggering 6.8 million tickets per hour were purchased in the waning hours leading up to the drawing yet only two people won! One of the two winners was from the small Arizona community of Fountain Hills. After announcing the winner's name, the local media was kind enough to show his house on the news so he'd be sure to bear the full burden of his sudden good fortune.

The medical marijuana dispensary lottery held on the morning of August 7, 2012, however, was different, as it held the very key to our future in the industry. Having to work at the pawn shop that day, I seriously doubted I'd be afforded the opportunity to tune in to the live online drawing broadcast by ADHS. In fact, I'd already come to peace with the reality that I wouldn't. Just in case, my co-worker Janice and I scrambled to locate a pair of speakers so we could hear what was being broadcast. Locating the speakers we spent another ten minutes trying to figure out how to plug the stupid things into the computer. All I can say is the stars must have been in alignment. I have no other explanation. For a period of no less than 45 minutes not a single, solitary person entered the normally busy shop. Not a one. Nor did anyone call on the phone. It was eerie, even conspiratorial.

At approximately 9:00 am or so a group of officials escorted lab-coat donning ADHS employees in front of a curtain. Patting themselves on the back, the state employees used phrases such as "what you're seeing here is only the tip of the iceberg" and "this is only 1% of the process, it took a team effort..." In reality, the lottery saved their bacon. The lottery replaced review criteria with pure, dumb luck.

After a mind-numbing explanation as to how the lottery would be administered (as if anyone didn't understand), numbered balls corresponding to each CHAA and applicant number were dumped out of hermetically-sealed plastic bags identified by officials as 'chain of custody bags' into a depression beneath the plastic hood of a large, upside-down clear-plastic salad bowl-like contraption with a vacuum tube sticking out the top. Ironically, the hermetically-sealed bags could easily have doubled as containers for transporting large quantities of medical-grade marijuana.

Beginning with the first CHAA and continuing on to the last, each hermetically-sealed bag was ceremoniously opened, ping pong balls dumped into the hopper. I honestly didn't think I was going to get nervous but as our CHAA number (20) drew near, the pacing began in earnest. As I mentioned earlier, nary a soul entered the pawn shop. Balls danced and floated as the air inside the salad bowl filled with cottony white orbs. After a period of about 18 or so *very long* seconds a man holding a stop watch released pressure on the vacuum allowing a ball to shoot to the surface. If your number was drawn you won. If it wasn't, that refund check for $1,000 would be in the mail...Eventually. For some odd reason I couldn't stop thinking that the late Don Ho, wherever he may be residing these days, would have been proud. I kept having flashbacks to his money-grabbing machine on Diamond Head where contestants struggled to grab as much cash as they could while bills blew around inside what looked like a phone booth.

My level of anxiety came to a crescendo as the two balls from CHAA 20 were deposited into the hopper. Our ball was marked 31. As for what the other ball was marked I can't recall. The balls floated around and around and around then with a final vacuum-sucking plop ball number 31 emerged at the top. Just like that we had won the lottery. Within minutes, my wife Phach and my dad, Ed 'Eddie' Quinn, called to offer condolences. Both had been cheering for a ball marked with the number 20 and so supposed we had lost the lottery. In all there were 97 (two of the 99 had been disputed before the drawing) dispensary registration certificates awarded that day from a pool of 404 applicants. Unfortunately, celebration was premature as the lottery drawing was merely the first step on a long and arduous trek.

Location, Location, Location

Wrapping up the application process had been a grind. Winning the lottery on the other hand had been pure luck. To our dismay, we soon discovered finding a viable location to house the dispensary would prove to be no picnic in the park. The unincorporated towns of Heber and Overgaard are diminutive with 90% of available commercial options straddling one side of Highway 260 or the other. The state of Arizona prohibits medical marijuana dispensaries from operating closer than 1000 feet from schools, day care facilities, parks, churches, and adult entertainment establishments (bars, strip clubs, pawn shops, etc.). While the state sets the guidelines, each municipality can enact its own, more stringent set of rules if it so pleases. As a business in an unincorporated sector, we were bound to the rules and regulations handed down by the county, which, in our particular case happened to be Navajo County. The county passed an ordinance extending the state's 1000-foot rule to 1500 feet. That might not sound like a big deal and it probably wouldn't be in a larger locale, but in the Heber-Overgaard area the extra 500 feet was a virtual death knell. There are three schools, a large park, too many churches to count, and several watering holes in the area. Every time we thought a location looked feasible, we found ourselves foiled by one of the aforementioned obstacles. One promising location was mere feet shy of the 1500-foot limit, as it was too close to the park. Another encouraging location sat too close to a church.

Making our way down the highway, we located a thousand-foot retail suite fitting our standards but found the owner reluctant and then wholly unwilling to lease the space to us. After turning us away with the excuse that the units had already been rented, the elderly female owner rented out one of the spaces to a church organization. Whether this was done in spite or borne from fear of prosecution is debatable. Jogging by occasionally on Sunday mornings, I've noticed the flock consists of three or four devout souls slumped heavily in folding card table chairs.

Though there are three other CHAAs in the county (Holbrook, Show Low, and Winslow), we were the only applicants dealing directly with the county for a special use permit, as the others dealt directly with their own city municipalities. The only way these others would be required to muddle through county bureaucracy was in the event they wanted to house a grow facility outside their city limits yet still inside the county line.

When it all seemed utterly hopeless, Dusty by a stroke of good fortune was able to find a new home for the dispensary. The building, consisting of four, 500-foot office suites, sat on the extreme eastern end of Overgaard. At the time one of the suites (located at one end of the plaza) was being rented out by a transportation company. Renting one and then quickly adding the other two available suites to our repertoire, we began remodeling in earnest. A new wood floor, fresh paint, additional walls and doors, pleather chairs – things were finally looking up. Or so we assumed.

~

Believing (quite naively in hindsight) that we were within a couple months of opening the doors on the new dispensary; we decided it was prudent to investigate one that was actually in operational mode. Problem was if we wanted to see one in operational mode, we'd have to travel to a state that actually had one operating. Bob Fern, leaps and bounds more sociable than either Dusty or myself, came across a woman named Tonya that owned a dispensary in Colorado Springs. To be honest, I have no idea where Bob came up with her number or how it all came about. All I knew was a week later we were piling into Bob's wife's Rav4 headed toward Colorado. Along for the ride were Bob, Dusty, my wife Phach, and her sulcata tortoise, Tortilla. I'd like to say the sights along the way were awe-inspiring, but as much of it traverses high, treeless plains, there isn't a whole lot for the mind to savor. Unless of course dilapidated billboards and bouncing tumbleweeds catch your fancy.

Only vaguely certain where the dispensaries we were scheduled to visit the following day were located, we opted for a Days Inn in what we were later told by locals was the 'ghetto side' of Colorado Springs. As we stood in the lobby waiting our turn to approach the counter, a couple of women engaged in a breezy fuss over the lack of cold AC in their room. The argument made little sense as it was mid-September and night-time temperatures were anything but balmy and at times downright chilly. If anything she should have been irate over a lack of heat. As I stood there listening to the woman's monologue my gaze happened on a sloppily written sign behind the counter announcing that the *Pool is close for Winter*. When I later brought the spelling gaff to the attention of the gruff, bovine-like woman manning the counter, she nonchalantly shot a quick glance over at the sign and exclaimed she saw no problem whatsoever. Why would she, she probably created the damn thing. Besides, what right had I, a simple lodger, to meddle in the proximity of an establishment's amenity with a time of year?

Since we were in town, Dusty and I decided it was a great opportunity to meet up with a few old friends for dinner so we arranged for Zeb Kettle, John 'Jav Sours' Sweet and his girlfriend, Amy Gillentine to meet us at the motel. Piling into two cars we headed over to old town Colorado Springs for a few pints, ribs, and laughs.

The next morning we headed over to Tonya's dispensary to see how things operated. Located in a defunct Walgreens (a detail I found acerbically sidesplitting), Tonya's place was tastefully laid out. Entering into a spacious waiting room, patients approached a glass window whereby they crammed their card underneath for approval. After consent from the window (these orifices are often bullet-proof), the patient entered a door (locked to the outside) leading into a modest room full of display cases containing jars of various medical marijuana products. Everything from prepackaged energy bars and elixirs to buds and kief (a resiny substance) were open to transaction. Joints were sold for as little as a couple bucks. When I referred to the items as such I was quickly brow-beaten, instructed that the items were known as 'pre-rolls' not joints. I suppose in some convention somewhere it was decided the term joint sounded too street-like and druggy whereas the word pre-roll had a much more medicinal and righteous ring to it. I found the notion absurd. I can go along with such things for a short walk down the primrose trial, but I do have my limits. What's more this line of reasoning falls completely to pieces when you realize that strains of medicinal-grade marijuana are assigned names such as Green Crack, Durban Poison, White Widow, Bubblicious, and AK-47.

We next visited the Tonya's grow facility tucked deep behind razor wire in a warehouse district alongside a cement factory. According to Colorado laws, each medical marijuana patient registering with a dispensary has a plant assigned to them. In theory, a dispensary grows a plant based on the number of patients on its rolls. Name tags and ID numbers are affixed to each plant. The system seems pretty hokey and perhaps has already changed in lieu of the new recreational legalization passed late last year.

After a bite to eat at a Mexican restaurant we headed to a combination dispensary/grow facility run by Tonya's friend William. Having taken over an entire shopping plaza, William, a bowtie enthusiast, was in the process of renovating and updating. The first thing I noted (to myself of course) was the need of a good exterminator as mice darted here and there among our feet as we toured the sprawling facility. William's claim to fame was a machine used to extract THC from his marijuana. An extract he used to create edible treats. Chief in charge of baking was an affable man named Gordon. Standing perhaps three and a half feet tall, Gordon had to crane his neck at an angle in order to peer up past the bill of his baseball cap when talking.

Whereas Arizona had limited the number of dispensaries to 126, Colorado had over twice that many in Denver alone. Colorado Springs had as many as 169 before new fees and regulations trimmed the number to around 70. With so many dispensaries vying for business, competition among each one obviously becomes keener. In order to get a leg up many outlets offer coupons and discounts. Some dispensaries go as far as employing sign-spinners wielding over-sized joints; I mean pre-rolls, as a way of enticing customers.

On the way home we decided to stay the night in Las Vegas, New Mexico. Once a stop on the Old West gambling circuit, it seems little has changed over the past century or so. One thing that had changed was the motel proprietors. Just like everywhere else in the country the sleeping establishments are now run by Indians (of the Asian variety) and Pakistanis. Pulling in at the Regal Motel, a genteel Indian man lacking most of his teeth handed over the keys to a couple of luxurious suites next to the ice machine.

In search of food, we soon found every restaurant in Las Vegas closed or in the process of closing. It was eight o'clock on a Saturday night. I can't imagine many comparisons are made between Las Vegas, New Mexico and its sin city cousin across the way in Nevada. After three or four unsuccessful attempts – one restaurant actually turned off their sign when we approached the front door – we finally found an Arby's with its lights on. Walking in I asked if they were still open and they tentatively nodded their heads. Finding this odd I asked what time they closed. 'Usually nine o'clock, but not always'. It was 8:08 pm. I felt like commenting that Doc Holliday would be rolling over in his grave upon discovering that the town, once notorious for its raucousness, rolled up the streets so early. But what was the use. The Arby's employees most likely had no idea who Doc Holliday was or the place in history their town held.

Though the entire motel was completely vacant, the manager/owner placed us right beside the only other occupants at the place – a trio of beer-swilling men sitting outside their room loudly conversing in Spanish well into the night. Needless to say I didn't sleep well that night.

As we made our way back to Arizona, we all felt content that the trip had been a worthy exploit. We had seen two successful (and operating) dispensaries and grow facilities. We had asked a lot of pertinent questions pertaining to day to day policies and procedures. We received what we thought were helpful tips. We also learned that banks wanted nothing to do with medical marijuana dispensaries as their ties to the FDIC might be jeopardized or worse yet the banks could be brought up on racketeering charges. At the moment it's strictly a cash and carry business reliant on strong safes and intricate security systems. Things are changing however. Recently the Justice Department and banking regulators have been hammering out plans to begin allowing legitimate marijuana-based businesses to open up bank accounts.

The next step in the journey was obtaining approval from the county in the form of a special use permit. To accomplish this we needed to attend a planning and zoning commission meeting and a board of supervisor's meeting. It gave the impression of being easily within reach. We had a competent team, a viable location, and a useful base of knowledge. What could possibly stop our progress?

A Transient Experience

A packed house confronted the planning and zoning board at the Holbrook Justice Center. Seated inconspicuously in the back row, I felt as if I was taking in an old colorized movie. A really, really bad old colorized movie...More precisely, a serious drama seen through my eyes as a farcical noir comedy. Caught in the clutches of paranoia and misinformation, one person after the next traipsed to the lectern to offer up grossly-biased, lop-sided opinions on why the county should deny us a special use permit for our dispensary. Though planning and zoning officials informed the gathering that the purpose of the meeting was not to debate the merits or evils of medical marijuana; instead to focus solely on the land usage issue at hand, the majority of the extremely one-sided discussion centered exclusively on the evils of devil weed without the slightest mention of the plant's medical capabilities.

Things appeared to go smoothly at the onset as Trent Larson from the county planning and zoning office offered a summary of our request followed up by a recommendation for the special use permit. Bob Fern followed Trent's summary up with a tactful speech of his own informing the crowd of our benevolent approach toward the patients of Navajo County. From that point on everything raced steadily downhill...

A dapper chap donning a tweed jacket was 'worried sick' about dispensary patients filling prescriptions before setting out for dazed walks down the walking path running through town. Exactly what it was that was supposed to happen on the walking path remains unknown? Stoned malfeasance? Public displays of nudity? Cannibalism? He never did say exactly. He just let the impression dangle there, allowing the partial bystanders to fill in their own scorecards.

Several residents of the Mogollon Airpark community directly across the highway from the proposed dispensary location raised safety concerns associated with the unregulated private runway servicing the neighborhood. The word *transient* was bandied about at least four or five times from four or five different residents giving rise to the notion the term had previously been rehearsed at a cocktail party. Whatever gave these people the notion that dispensary patients were transients I never could figure out? Were they alluding to the word transient in the manner of walking the earth nomadically or transient in the manner of site-based homelessness? In any event, their fears seemed to concern transients leaving the dispensary in a dazed state and walking about aimlessly on the runway directly into the oncoming path of an approaching Cessna. I can't begin to explain how hard it was to sit back and listen to what I was hearing. Biting hard on my tongue, I wanted to jump up and explain the expense attached to medical-grade marijuana. I wanted to assure them transients were the least of their worries, as medical marijuana is certainly not affordable on just any bum's budget. Furthermore, the state strictly forbade loitering or smoking marijuana on the premises. This wasn't a marijuana public house, it was a marijuana pharmacy. Even though all of this had been explained in detail at the beginning of the meeting it obviously hadn't sunk in. Furthermore, it was never going to.

Curiously, the Town Manager of Taylor (a neighboring town) made the trek over to put his two cents in regarding the special use permit. The rather rotund man led off his discourse by saying 'Well I figure it's gonna happen in Taylor sometime soon too...' He obviously hadn't received the memo. There would be no dispensary in Taylor so long as there was one in Overgaard as the two towns were in the same CHAA and only one dispensary was permitted per CHAA.

Let me be honest, there are quite a few businesses I wouldn't want popping up next to my home or business...A bar, nightclub, strip joint...Therefore, I could understand the initial apprehension of the couple running the body shop business directly next door to the proposed dispensary. They were worried people might shy away from bringing their cars in for paint jobs due to the close proximity of the dispensary. They complained that their children would be at risk after school when the bus dropped them off. Risk from exactly what or who wasn't fully expounded...A ghoulish cancer patient in a trench coat enticingly offering joints to third graders? Besides, we're talking about a body shop here full of paint fumes, air tools, sand blasters, and spark-emitting grinders. Not exactly what I would consider a safe environment for kids. Let's pretend for the sake of argument I was a single parent who happened to work at a steel mill. I'm low on cash and don't really trust others watching my kids after school. So, with this in mind, I make arrangements to have the school bus drop my kids off at the steel mill after school. My children run around and entertain themselves at the mill until the whistle blows. 'Be careful around that hot cauldron sweetie.' Scary thought isn't it. On the verge of tears, the body shop man pleaded with the board to nix our application saying he would have never opened up a business next to a 'pot house' (sniffle, sniffle) had he known one was going in. From that day on the body shop man has been referred to simply as the "Cry Baby".

As the hours rolled on, it became abundantly apparent we would receive a denial from the board. We did. Unanimously. Although zoning concerns had all checked out positively, we were considered a safety threat to the community. Ghouls, goblins, zombies, and lest we not forget…Transients.

By a Camel's Nose...BOS I

I would like to report that the Board of Supervisor's meeting was in some way different from the previously mentioned Planning and Zoning meeting. But it wasn't. In fact, if anything it was worse. Had our expectations been too high? It seemed inconceivable that the board would deny us a permit given that the program had been sanctioned by the state and the proposed building zoned 100% compliant. As at the previous meeting, Dusty, Bob, and I were the lone supporting cast. This time around I was to speak on our behalf. Armed with notecards at the ready, I sat patiently as Homero Vela from planning and zoning led off with a strong presentation. Just like the previous meeting, a recommendation for the special use permit was offered. Although Homero stole most of my material, I felt confident we would receive the go ahead after explaining we were analogous to a pharmacy and obligated to follow the laws and guidelines set down by the state. I illustrated through words that our dispensary would be run by a group of professionals in a professional manner in strict adherence to the law. I attempted to bang home our desire to work with and be an integral part of the community.

No sooner had I taken my seat that it all came crashing down as one member of the opposition after the next, perhaps thirty in all, made his or her way to the dais intent on striking a blow against marijuana. There were no exceptions made for medicinal purposes. As for a discussion involving to zoning issues, which as to my understanding was the very essence of the special use permit, there was none.

One staunch advocate made a lavish speech in the defense and well-being of the airpark runway. Ranting and raving, he wondered aloud what might happen if a dispensary customer ran amok after leaving the shop in a daze of glory (my words). 'What if after their sixth joint a person mistook the runway for Highway 260?' (His words) Six joints? Really? Remember we're talking about medicinal quality marijuana not Mexican pack weed. I don't even think Snoop Dogg could pull off smoking six joints in a row. Moreover, the comment came after I had just finished explaining that loitering wasn't an option as the state doesn't allow it and neither would the dispensary. Why would we want people hanging around getting high in our parking lot? Do people fill prescriptions at Walgreens and dose up in the parking lot for kicks before driving home? The entire argument was baseless and meaningless.

One after the next, concerned and clearly outraged citizens shuffled up to the microphone. Each new speaker carried along with them sound bites of disinformation. The prevailing theme centered squarely upon the 'moral breakdown in the fiber of society'. There was rough talk of killing sprees and violent beatings meted out by crazed drug addicts. I couldn't shake eerie images from the films *Billy Jack* and *Alice's Restaurant* from my head for nearly a week.

A man voiced distress over the inherent possibility of intoxicated drivers running roughshod through town. 'If they produce a card [state-issued medical marijuana card] our hands are tied, there is nothing we can do. At .04 a person can be deemed drunk, but with weed there is nothing that can be done…' Like most of the gibberish from the peanut gallery, the man had no idea what he was talking about. First of all the state limit for driving while under the influence is .08 not .04. Secondly, a person most certainly can be charged for driving under the influence if found to be under the influence of marijuana. Or cocaine. Or even fatigue.

A haranguing woman warned the board there wouldn't be enough security to deter customers from 'selling drugs the minute they walked out of the building.' I wanted to ask if this would occur before or after they moseyed up the road to the airstrip.

The following was one of my favorite lines of the day: 'It's like a camel puttin' his head in the tent.' I knew straight away what the woman was referring to but I'd be willing to bet many in the audience were confused as she gave no explanation to her comment. Where was Barry Goldwater when we needed him? Goldwater famously used the adage on the senate floor in 1958 when referring to a piece of legislation. I did some research on the origin of the Arabic phrase and found it traced back to 1858.

The Camel's Nose In The Tent!

One cold night, as an Arab sat in his tent, a camel gently thrust his nose under the flap and looked in. "Master," he said, "let me put my nose in your tent. It's cold and stormy out here." "By all means," said the Arab, "and welcome" as he turned over and went to sleep.

A little later the Arab awoke to find that the camel had not only put his nose in the tent but his head and neck also. The camel, who had been turning his head from side to side, said, "I will take but little more room if I place my forelegs within the tent. It is difficult standing out here." "Yes, you may put your forelegs within," said the Arab, moving a little to make room, for the tent was small.

Finally, the camel said, "May I not stand wholly inside? I keep the tent open by standing as I do." "Yes, yes," said the Arab. "Come wholly inside. Perhaps it will be better for both of us." So the camel crowded in. The Arab with difficulty in the crowded quarters again went to sleep. When he woke up the next time, he was outside in the cold and the camel had the tent to himself.

Author unknown

"If the camel once gets his nose in the tent, his body will soon follow." *Old Arabian proverb*

The basic premise here…God help us once marijuana gets its foot in the door and a firm hold on society. One thing will lead to another. The slope will become slippery as the dominoes fall one after the next. As the Chinese say, *de long wang shu*, which roughly translates to the old English adage: *Give them an inch; they'll take a mile.*
One woman, shaking her fists in the air (I'm not making this stuff up), insisted we produce a business plan. 'I wanna see the business plan!' 'I wanna know how much money they can make!' Homero attempted to pacify her by explaining that businesses are not required to offer business plans when applying for special use permits. He explained not even almighty

Wal Mart would be asked to do so. 'Why don't they just sell the stuff at Walgreens', railed the woman. 'I don't get it, if it is so important to *these* people why don't they just get it at the pharmacy?' We explained that FDA regulations precluded medical marijuana from being sold and distributed at pharmacies but I don't really think it sunk in judging by her follow up comment as to whether marijuana would be covered under Obamacare.

The Overgaard Chamber of Commerce president announced a full 90% of the businesses in the Heber-Overgaard area stood in opposition to the dispensary. Failing to adequately explain why this was so, she seethed and wriggled as if the devil had possessed her.

The drubbing continued for two hours before the board mercifully called a recess to convene in quarters – a back room somewhere filled with cheese whiz and potato chips. Not one solitary thing had been queried regarding our operations. There were no enquiries as to how we acquired product. No questions pertaining to growing marijuana or how much we intended to harvest. Sated from their snacks – orange crumbs dusted the front of one board member's shirt – the board returned after twenty-five minutes or so to render its verdict. The tally: 4-1 in opposition. Our special use permit had been denied. Only one member, the chair, had voted in our favor, 'not because he liked the idea, but because he had taken an oath to uphold state laws'. Once again It all boiled down to the 'safety of the community', a nebulous phrase and concept left completely undefined. A phrase left dangling in the air like those lottery balls several months earlier. In the end, it was widely apparent that safety wasn't really the issue; people just hated the idea of a dispensary in their town. *Anywhere but Here* and *Not in our Backyard* were prevailing slogans.

Feeling low that evening I walked over to the airpark runway in search of stoned-out zombies and transient souls lurking about. Low and behold I came across several pairs of gray-haired strollers out for a saunter. Oblivious to any safety concerns, the couples walked directly down the middle of the runway.

The very next day I began putting together a letter to the board. A plea if you will. It was the only plan of action we could think of in lieu of contacting lawyers and bringing lawsuits. Judging from the tone of the planning and zoning and board of supervisor meetings neither the board nor the community grasped the ramifications involved with denying our dispensary an opportunity to open in Overgaard. The following is the final version of the letter sent out to the board members. My earlier versions were much more entertaining but Heather found my tone overly satirical so I agreed in the best interests of the business to water down my comments and thoughts. To this day I'm not sure whether the board members read the letter or not as to my knowledge we never received any sort of reply or comment. We did however manage to wrangle a meeting with the supervisor assigned to our district.

December 4, 2012

What's Really In The Best Interest Of The Community?

Upon leaving the Board of Supervisor's Meeting on Tuesday (November 27), we all felt a deep disconnect among the public's distinction between a state-regulated medical marijuana dispensary and home grows currently being conducted and marijuana compassion clubs/consultation centers entering the area. They seem to misunderstand that it is more desirable and safer for the community to continue to allow people to grow marijuana in their homes completely unregulated.

There are many Heber-Overgaard residents, professionals, business owners, planning & zoning, sheriff deputies, firemen, and parishioners whom are all educated on the difference between a dispensary which is state-regulated versus home growers that are not regulated and being abused. Some residents of the community present at the meeting want to continue allowing local marijuana card holders and others to grow marijuana in their homes without regulation by the state laws of Arizona. We spoke to many of these residents who understand we want to provide service in accordance with the state regulated guidelines and in favor of our dispensary. Does the community truly understand the dangers involved with home grown setups? The plants are grown using multiple high-intensity lights, which have the potential of becoming extremely flammable when not vented or wired correctly. They are not getting permits or licensed contractors when setting up these so called unregulated grow rooms which pose a threat to nearby neighbors should a fire arise due to negligence. When someone learns of a home grow, there is bound to be more traffic and criminal activity in the local neighborhoods and violent home invasions are possible.

Another concern is what are these home growers doing with all the "extra" marijuana they are growing? A caregiver can currently grow up to 72 plants at any one time. Where does this "extra", unregulated marijuana end up? At one of the many compassion clubs that continue to operate until a local dispensary shuts them down. We have recently been approached with many inquiries and a state-wide cannabis club vendor in regards to subletting our proposed dispensary site with the intention of establishing a compassion club/medical marijuana center. We have also heard rumors that other sites in both Heber and Overgaard are also being discussed. *Mountain Meds* and *Nature's Harvest* are businesses located in the Pinetop-Lakeside area. These businesses currently function as consultation or compassion clubs distributing medical marijuana to area cardholders. Without a dispensary in the Heber-Overgaard/Snowflake-Taylor CHAA, these businesses will soon move into our area, which have now taken over the Phoenix Metro Area and do not require special use permits to operate.

We at Overgaard Compassion Care stand opposed to compassion clubs! Dispensaries are regulated by state statute, compassion clubs are not! Compassion clubs encourage marijuana leaves and bold signage, unsightly banners that advertise on the entire face of the buildings. Human sign spinners will attract the many who pass or drive by. Caregivers are also considering moving into the area since the Glendale dispensary has now opened and the home growers will be forced to shut down. Do we really want a rush of unqualified growers moving into our area with the specific intent of growing marijuana and opening up compassion clubs in a wide-open CHAA free from the absence of a state regulated dispensary?

Overgaard Compassion Care has carefully abided by and followed all the stringent guidelines that the state and county has mandated in order to move us safely to the next step. The sheriff's department, planning & zoning as

113

well as the local fire department would much rather have one professional grow room that meets all county building codes operating in town rather than hundreds of unprofessional, unregulated, non-zoned compliant grows that are going on in households. We are all in agreement that having unregulated fashionable compassion clubs that will flood our quiet community in the next couple months without any way to stop them before they start. As community leaders wouldn't everyone agree to put up with a discreet, state-mandated, professionally-run, highly-regulated medical marijuana dispensary than unregulated marijuana compassion clubs and home grows?

At this time in order to move forward on this issue if we cannot come to a mutual agreement, we will consider legal counsel as a last resort. We would much rather work on a friendly basis with the Board, the county, and the community to resolve these issues. We would like to schedule an appointment as soon as possible to meet face to face at your offices to discuss these issues personally. Thank you again for taking the time to read our letter of concerns.

Sincerely,

Overgaard Compassion Care

A Face to Face with the Super

*A*s I mentioned at the tail end of the previous chapter in a last ditch effort to avoid hiring a law firm, we felt it wise to pursue a meeting with one of the three dissenting supervisors whom had voted against us at the Navajo County Board of Supervisor's meeting on 11-27-12. We expected the meeting to be a waste of time and in the end…It pretty much was. Then I don't know precisely what we were expecting. The man is deeply set in his ways and doesn't give a damn what we (or anyone else for that matter) thinks or says. Nor did he give a damn what a judge in Phoenix thought about medical marijuana. Producing a photocopy of a newspaper article from that day's *Arizona Republic*, I showed him the ruling by Judge Gordon in a case comparable to our own. The White Mountain group had been denied a special use permit from Maricopa County for a prospective dispensary location in Sun City. Analogous to our sticky situation, Sun City similarly falls under the jurisdiction of a county and not a municipality. Maricopa County Attorney Bill Montgomery had taken up a personal crusade to snuff out medical marijuana in the state of Arizona. Montgomery later went down in flames in the appellate court during appeal. Here is the *Arizona Republic* article dated December 5, 2012:

Arizona's medical marijuana law is constitutional and federal drug laws don't stand in the way of public officials implementing the state law, a judge ruled Tuesday. "This court will not rule that Arizona, having sided with the ever-growing minority of states and having limited it to medical use, has violated public policy," Judge Michael Gordon of Maricopa County Superior Court wrote. The case started over a dispute whether Maricopa County had to approve zoning for a dispensary in Sun City. It grew to include the larger legal question of whether federal drug laws pre-empt Arizona's medical marijuana law. Under Gordon's ruling, county officials must provide the White Mountain Health Center with documentation that it complies with local zoning restrictions. During an Oct. 19 hearing, attorneys for the American Civil Liberties Union and its Arizona affiliate argued that the Arizona law is not pre-empted by federal drug laws. They said the state is allowed to make policy decisions on medical marijuana. Lawyers for the state Attorney General's Office and Maricopa County argued that the state's medical marijuana law cannot be fully implemented because federal drug laws make it a crime to possess, grow or distribute marijuana and because federal laws are considered supreme over state statutes. Arizona allows use of medical marijuana for such conditions as cancer, chronic pain and muscle spasms. Arizona health officials have started licensing the first dispensaries in the state, and the first one is expected to open with days. More than 30,000 people already have cards authorizing them to possess and use medical marijuana. Most of those people also had authorizations to grow marijuana, but those authorizations get phased out once a dispensary is licensed in their area and once their card with current growing authorizing comes up for renewal annually. County Attorney Bill Montgomery told Gordon during the Oct. 19 hearing that county employees could face prosecution by the federal government for aiding and abetting drug crimes if the dispensaries open, while ACLU attorney Ezekiel Edwards said government workers really aren't at risk of prosecution. White Mountain Health Center sued the county after it rejected the facility's registration certificate, which is part of the state requirement to become a medical-marijuana dispensary applicant. The case took on broader focus when Montgomery and Attorney General Tom Horne made separate but coordinated requests in the court case, specifically targeting the Arizona law's dispensary provisions. Gordon had already ruled that state health officials could not decline to award a dispensary license to White Mountain because of the county's inaction, but Horne and Montgomery asked the judge to dismiss White Mountain's lawsuit on grounds that Arizona's law is illegal. Horne and Republican Gov. Jan Brewer previously asked a federal judge to rule on whether Arizona's law is pre-empted. However, the judge refused, ruling in January that the state officials hadn't established a genuine threat of prosecution of state employees for administering the law. Also last January, a state trial judge ordered the state to proceed with allowing creation of dispensaries and lifted some of the state's restrictions [namely residency requirements].The state has issued use and growing permits to thousands of individuals, but Brewer for months balked at implementing the dispensary part of the law.

The supervisor snuffled his nose, at least I think that's what it was anyway, and said he didn't 'care what one judge said'. 'About anything.' Entering into a blustery tirade, the supervisor explained how a judge had ruined his family's business over a 'stupid spotted owl'. I carefully explained that Judge Gordon's decision had dismissed the threat of Federal interference as a basis for denial (something that the supervisor had used as an excuse earlier) but he didn't want to hear about it.

One of the county planners who had so bravely and craftily had our back at the previous two meetings at the county complex seemed to have lost his enthusiasm. Another county planner, the number one man at the planning and zoning office, attempted to debate (albeit tenderly) with the supervisor on technical merit but soon straightened out his act as well. I was confused as to why they were even there. It wasn't like the supervisor needed any cheerleaders and surely needed no reinforcement.

'When the Navajos voted against the special use permit I knew it didn't matter anymore because that split the vote,' said the supervisor. One supervisor had called in sick leaving only four at the meeting. The supervisor, alternately referring to the two Navajo Board Members as 'natives', acknowledged my sentiments that the Navajos had no vested interest in the permit. I didn't go as far as saying they shouldn't *have had* a vote on the matter, but my undertone must have belied as much. One of the planners was quick to jump to the Indians side by sermonizing that the tribe played a monumental role in the county. At a different setting – perhaps at a bar or picnic – I might have belabored the point but dismissed it as pointless at that particular juncture. How can Indians on reservations consider themselves sovereign yet still be allowed to participate in county affairs? This doesn't seem right to me at all. The supervisor went on to assert that the 'natives' were against all things marijuana because of the ill effects found on the Navajo Reservation. It was my turn to snuffle. 'Problems', I said with a sneer. 'That's quite an understatement.' The supervisor offered a sly, telling sneer of his own knowing damn well he hadn't a leg to stand on when it came to the status quo found on the reservation.

You'll recall at the Board of Supervisor's meeting an Overgaard resident had stood up at the dais and asked what would happen if a person purchasing medical marijuana at our dispensary smoked six joints and then confused the highway for the runway. I asked the supervisor if the six-joint fairy tale had influenced his opinion in any way. Bug snort again. 'Please...Are you asking me if I believe people are going to get stoned and catch a face full of propeller? 'Our decision was based purely on the law not on those crazy comments.' If it were based purely on the law he would have voted in our favor. After all, the state had given its blessing. But his decision had been based *purely* on his opinion.

As the meeting disintegrated, the supervisor smugly inquired whether we were making improvements on the property. We acknowledged we had been making a few minor changes. Snuffle. 'Not what I hear, my nephew was on the crew down there. I understand there was a complaint filed against the body shop the very next day after the board shot down your special use permit. Sounds a little vindictive to me.' I explained there were two or three sides to every story but again, the man wasn't listening.

Leaving the meeting, Dusty summed up the supervisor's demeanor to a T. The man is eerily reminiscent of the antagonistic county bigwig, Jefferson Davis 'J.D.' Hogg on the television series *The Dukes of Hazzard*. Unfortunately there weren't any Daisy Dukes or hot rod cars to lighten up the mood. He reminded us again and again how unwilling he was to sacrifice his principles by allowing such a dastardly thing as a medical marijuana dispensary to operate on *his* turf.

As I alluded to earlier, the meeting had pretty much been a waste of everyone's time. There was talk of compromise but there was really nothing to compromise as we had no other plots of land. Even if there was a plot available we hadn't the money to buy it. Besides, building permits and construction timelines would never have worked as we only had six months to obtain the operating license. The supervisor wasn't about to back down. He stood on principle. He told us it had been hard to decide but he was clearly bullshitting. The decision to deny the permit had been easy for him. It gave him a rush. A sense of power.

Lawyers

*A*fter our dismal meeting with the supervisor it became abundantly apparent we needed legal counsel of some species to carry on the fight. Feeling we were being discriminated unfairly I wrote letters to various lawyers attaching themselves to NORML (National Organization for the Reform of Marijuana Laws) but received no response. I did eventually hear back (after repeated letters) from a spokesman from the organization informing me: 'NORML is a lobby for marijuana smokers, not an industry lobby. So we are probably not the right group to fight your fight. There are industry groups at both the national and state level, and I would expect they might want to help you.' They apparently didn't as repeated efforts remained fruitless. Next, I contacted the law college at Arizona State University in hopes that an ambitious law student might take up the cause. None did. I then contacted the ACLU, which did respond – eight or nine weeks later – calling to see how things were going. Of course by then we had already hired a lawyer and were in discussions with the county concerning another Board of Supervisor's meeting. Our pro bono options seemed to be withering away.

Leaving the icy temperatures of northeastern Arizona behind us in the rearview mirror, Dusty and I ventured down the escarpment for a meeting with Scottsdale-based lawyer, Jeffrey Kaufman. Kaufman had recently made headlines for his work with a dispensary being snubbed by the powers that be in Maricopa County so we knew he had a working knowledge of medical marijuana. The meeting in Kaufman's office was akin to being transported to an earlier era – 1979 to be precise. Cardboard boxes competed for floor space with outmoded chairs and passé end tables exhibiting plastic plants which had originally been green but are now white with dandruff-like dust. Behind a cluttered desk sat Kaufman, charming and affable in a cheap blue suit of a vintage paralleling the other fixtures in the room. Despite the look and feel of the place I felt comfortable. Kaufman didn't seem to emit that aura of smugness often exuded by members of his self-exalted clan. Bob Fern had driven over from his home in Chandler and Heather joined in on the fun via speaker phone from Ohio. The meeting, lasting about an hour, went well. We informed Kaufman we'd get back to him very soon.

Several days later we headed down the escarpment once again, this time to the offices of the Rose Law Group. Like the meeting with Kaufman, Bob drove over from Chandler and Heather tuned in via speaker phone. We were assigned an attorney named H. Ryan Hurley who, like Kaufman, was familiar with medical marijuana legislation. The contents of the meeting were identical…What could be done about opening up our dispensary? How soon could we bring a lawsuit? What could we hope to gain? The same questions we had already posed to Kaufman. Both lawyers had said that all options with the county must be exercised and exhausted before bringing a lawsuit. If not a judge would simply toss any lawsuit out. At the conclusion of the meeting Dusty handed a wad of bills to Hurley and our saga with lawyers commenced. Had it been up to me I probably would have went with Kaufman. Heather, holding the silver, felt the Rose Law firm possessed the best reputation so we went with Hurley. It was yet to be determined whether a snazzy office filled with expensive accoutrements and a fancy glass table equated to a competent legal team. Requiring a $10,000 retainer, Hurley said he'd write a scare letter to the county threatening to sue. A tactic we were hoping to avoid as suing was not only costly but far from a sure bet, especially given that a board member's uncle or nephew could quite possibly be the judge of record.

Winter of *Our* Discontent

*D*ays became weeks. Weeks became months. Snowstorms came and went leaving arctic air in their wake. The dispensary grand opening, optimistically thought to arrive by early January, was still nowhere on the foreseeable horizon. Everything seemed to bog down as if in slow motion. This period of inactivity was exceptionally difficult on Dusty and Phach. As an eremitic, I have little trouble entertaining myself by running and watching sports. By reading and writing. Reading Paul Theroux's *Ghost Train to the Eastern Star* I came across a paragraph that concisely summed up the feelings I had at the time I was working on this chapter. Speaking of a dinner party and the possibility of meeting a Turkish writer named Orhan Pamuk, Theroux writes:

'...I was eager to meet him, not merely because of his well-made novels and his personal history in *Istanbul*, but because, as a passionate writer and self-described graphomaniac, he was probably eccentric, someone who lived at the edge of the world, the solitary soul that all writers must be in order to do their work and live their lives. Writers are always readers, and though they are usually unbalanced, they are always noticers of the world.'

Though I must admit there was somewhat of a disadvantage to my fallback on reading as it made me yearn for travel and the escapes such undertakings offer. I've never been one longing for daily social visitations filled with drab, mindless prattle. When a personal need for socialization arises, I cure what ails me by basking in an overloaded state of mass confusion through frenetic dashes into crowded, impossible spaces. The clash and clattering of human engrossment entices my senses. The more diverse and more chaotic the better. Preferably in a third world country. I don't fear crowds I just don't care much for them. I do, however, enjoy watching from the sidelines…The ballet, the symphonic orchestrations of strained movement and interaction. When I get my fill, when I'm satiated, I retreat once more into a boring yet satisfying existence of conciliatory solitude. But I do understand this hunger for civilization and human contact. I really do. I'm an anomaly. I'm not typical. Many people crave social contact. Modern conveniences. Fast food restaurants. Movie theaters. Starbucks. The things I most miss about the city aside from visiting friends and family are playing soccer and attending Arizona Diamondback's baseball games.

Our days at this juncture mainly involved working at the shop in the unlikely event we received a call from the lawyers informing us that the county had capitulated by handing down a special use permit. Every month the doors remained closed meant paying rent and utilities on three office spaces generating a grand total of zero dollars. Judging by the lawn chairs circling the blackened fire pit behind the complex, the only ones getting any use out of the place was the landlord's brother Brian and his assistant EB.

Diversions and digressions

Just as Phach and I were pulling into the Holbrook DMV parking lot Dusty called with the news that he had incurred yet another bout with an ornery kidney stone which had required him to catch a ride in a bologna wagon (ambulance) from Overgaard over to the nearest hospital in Show Low. A distance of over 40 miles. I told Dusty that Phach was just about to take the road test for her driver's license and that we'd head out for Show Low to pick him up as soon as she was finished. Upon snapping my phone shut and walking up to the door, I discovered that the DMV office was closed for lunch. Worse yet there were three or four carloads of people waiting to storm the lobby the minute it reopened at one pm. Phach would have to wait another day or two.

After a one-hour drive through the high plains to Show Low we found Dusty waiting uncomfortably in the lobby. An MRI had revealed a 5 mm kidney stone lodged in his bladder. Doctors told him there was nothing to do but wait for the large impediment to either dissolve or shoot the rapids through his innards. A few weeks later Dusty had yet another attack and yet another ride in an ambulance. This time around a stent was slipped up his privates and the impediment removed by means of a surgical procedure. I don't recall seeing anyone in so much pain and agony. It makes me want to gulp down a gallon of water just thinking about it. When I had dropped Dusty off at the fire station for the ambulance ride to Show Low he was unaware of anything but intense pain, nodding in and out of consciousness as firemen poked and prodded at him as they attempted to prompt a response. He later told me he had absolutely no recollection of any pokings or proddings.

The following morning Phach and I made the 40-mile jaunt over to Holbrook for another shot at the license. After filling out a form a woman told Phach to meet her out by the parallel parking area located adjacent to the tumble-down shack passing for the DMV office. The woman graciously offered a drawing explaining what was expected. 'You get three tries to pass the test. But you only have to successfully parallel park one time. But if you hit the cones then you're finished and you have to come back on a different day. Do you understand?' Phach shook her head in the affirmative while I pointed to the drawing and explained to the woman that Phach wouldn't have to worry about hitting any cones because they were on top of the roof. The woman looked at me as if I were a crackpot and went about her business. You see, when we had pulled into the parking lot that morning I noticed the parallel parking cones sitting up on top of the DMV building's roof. I admit it didn't make much sense but then many things I encounter don't. Unable to draw a feasible explanation, I assumed the DMV personnel had a bureaucratic, if not completely logical reason for the cones being on the roof. Perhaps by throwing the cones on the roof each night they considered them safe from theft? I imagined an employee fishing each orange cone one by one off the roof each morning with a long pole such as those used to clean swimming pools.

Improvising, I took one of the sawhorses out of the back of my dad's jeep so Phach could practice before the employee came out to test her. Ten minutes later the woman came outside. The look on her face was priceless.

'What happened to the cones?'

'I told you, they were up on the roof.'

Puzzled, she came around the corner and took a look for herself. 'They are up on the roof!' 'I thought you were kidding!'

I didn't say this of course, but sure as hell was thinking it…Why would I make a joke about cones being on the roof? As we stood discussing the sordid details of the cones-on-the-roof-mystery Phach executed a perfect parallel parking job around the sawhorse. The woman, still flabbergasted over the cones being on the roof, exclaimed 'I guess you pass!' The employee said she had personally placed the cones out an hour earlier and had no idea how they could have wound up on the roof.

A few minutes later a second DMV employee, this one bundled up in a bright orange jacket favored by highway workers along the ALCAN Highway jumped into the jeep's passenger seat for the road test. I was curious as to the jacket's purpose. Was it standard operating procedure in case of breakdown during the road test?

I stood outside and waited for their return. I didn't have to wait long. Five minutes later the jeep was pulling back into the parking lot. Phach had passed. Apparently the woman, coughing and sneezing, only had Phach drive a few blocks down the way into a trailer park and back. Here we had wasted our time and gas driving the 40 mile route to Holbrook on three separate occasions to practice making turns in the lighted intersections (there are only three traffic lights in Holbrook but none in the town of Overgaard where we live).

~

Back at the dispensary we continued to ready the facility by completing necessary tasks, but mainly what we did was a lot of waiting. We waited for phone calls from lawyers that never came. We waited for county officials to get back with us. During this period of interminable waiting, I found it reassuring to watch a program called *Bering Sea Gold*. Much like its predecessors and contemporaries *Bering Sea Gold* is a reality television show based on gold. While I ashamedly admit enjoying many of the gold shows (*Gold Rush, Bamazon, Jungle Gold*, etc.) it was *Bering Sea Gold* that I most identified with – both the hopefulness and hopelessness of dredging for gold off the coast of Nome, Alaska. Eccentrics and misfits trying their best to succeed against all odds. Some live in shacks, some in rusty old trailers. Others eke out existences in tents anchored down by rocks on windswept beaches. I live in an old trailer produced a year before Woodstock, New York became a household name. Nights are frigid and there is no money in the coffers to run the propane heater. Like the coal tender on a steam engine, I constantly shovel wood into the wood-burning stove. It isn't hard to see why I so easily identify with the schleps on the show. Yet it wasn't only the harsh living that identified with. It was the make it or break it reality confronting me. Instead of gold or bust, it was weed or bust.

February brought with it yet another diversion. The annual pig hunt. Nearly every February for the past twenty-five years I've made the trip over to Congress, Arizona to hunt javelina. What began as a small group has blossomed into a very large gathering. What formerly was three or four days of hard hunting and partying has transformed over the years into lighter hunting and harder partying as fewer and fewer each year seem to actually possess tags for hunting, coming instead for the revelry. While hunting pigs with a large revolver is a blast, the thing I like most about attending the quasi-reunion is to reunite with old friends. An opportunity to catch up, as it is oftentimes the only chance I get to see most of the people in attendance as they live in Phoenix and I no longer do. What used to be a snappy, leisurely, one-hour drive now takes me five as there is no efficient way to access the location from the where I live on the Mogollon Rim. Descending the rim to Payson I have to ascend it once more before descending down a long final stretch to the Verde Valley. Though it is shorter to take I-17 south a ways then over to Prescott, I normally stop off along the way to visit my old friend Jeff 'Clarence' Linssen at his shop, Inxon Tattoo In Cottonwood. After visiting a few hours I make my way through the artsy town of Jerome, a former gold mining enclave before topping off on Mingus Mountain. From there it is downhill to Prescott Valley and Prescott where traffic has become citified over the years as more and more people have moved in from places such as California. Progressing onward through the towns of Nowhere (I'm not making this up) and Skull Valley, I gas up in Peeples Valley before plunging down Yarnell Hill to Congress.

  With an elevation of over 3,000 feet the weather in early February is a mixed bag in the high desert. It can be cool or warm bordering on hot. Some years it is extremely dry while others it is extremely wet. This particular year it was windy and cool bordering on windy and cold with a rare snowstorm dropping a few inches on our camp the second night out. As the only hunter hailing from the mountainous and snowy regions of Arizona I was the lone dissenter of this snow excitement, retiring to my tent as the others played like children making snowballs and frolicking. This gamboling in the wet flakes was gravely dampened when Howard Hughes' grandson Cale accidently ate a corn chip containing peanuts sending him into anaphylactic shock. Though Howard administered a medicinal plunger, erring on the side of caution the pair made haste to the Congress Fire Department where an awaiting ambulance transported Cale to the Wickenburg Hospital, Howard following behind in his truck. Cale was fine but Howard, in his cups and not expecting to drive anywhere, narrowly sidestepped DUI checkpoints erected to ensnare merrymakers at a rodeo being held in Wickenburg. The roadblocks were set up on the south side of town restricting rodeo-goers en route to Phoenix. Fortunately for Howard, authorities didn't seem all that concerned with those headed north.

Ron Guy was the lone hunter to shoot a pig. Stuffing the good-sized critter into a pit filled with fiery coals we played horseshoes and drank beer, reminiscing about past hunts and catching up. Four days later I was back home. Still waiting. We had yet to hear anything from our lawyers.

Fun and Games in Holbrook...BOS II

*I*t became obvious that the intimidation letter penned by our attorneys failed to produce much of a fright as county officials didn't even bother returning correspondence with our high-dollar legal team. Tired of waiting, we were ready to push forward with a lawsuit. The clock was ticking. We only had until June 7th (2013) to complete the operational component of our dispensary license. Without the special use permit from the county we had no chance of ever opening. Suing for the special use permit seemed our only option. Our lawyer, however, seemed hesitant to move forward with the lawsuit focusing instead on ways to sway the county. The specifics of any banter between Hurley and the county (had there been any) were obscure, as a deep gulf of non-communication existed between our team and the lawyers. It was common for the law firm to rack up billing statements to the tune of $305 dollars an hour for 'discussing' or 'reviewing' the case but we rarely if ever received updates without begging for them. If it sounds like I have a bad taste in my mouth for lawyers it's because I do. In the midst of this indecisiveness by Hurley and company we received a curious email from Trent Larson down at Navajo County Planning and Zoning. Apparently someone at the county suggested our case be brought back to a second Board of Supervisor's Meeting. As to who suggested rehearing the case I'm still not sure. Had the county attorney mulled over the scare letter from the lawyers and decided to let the issue be heard again? In the interval since the previous meeting two new board members had been sworn in. I wasn't sure whether that was good news or not but since the vote had been nearly unanimous against us the first go round, I surmised it couldn't get much worse.

In preparation for the latest board meeting we decided it was prudent to reach out to the community. Scheduling time down at the county community center, we invited the public to an informational meeting concerning medical marijuana and the specifics of our proposed dispensary. Creating a PowerPoint presentation for the occasion, Dusty and I arrived twenty minutes early to set things up and wait for an audience. Two minutes before the scheduled meeting time the husband and wife local newspaper team arrived. Five minutes later (and three minutes late) Dusty's neighbor Cindy and her nephew arrived. They only attended because Dusty had urged them to attend and besides, they didn't have anything else going on. A man named Craig, whom Bob Fern had encouraged to attend, arrived minutes later. No one else showed up. If you ask me, the meeting had been boycotted. This theory seemed to be backed up by the fact that a large gathering amassed several hours later at the chamber of commerce. The hot topic on tap: The medical marijuana dispensary threatening to devour our idyllic community. I presented the slideshow – one that had taken several hours to produce – and fielded questions from the meager attendance. The newspaper people were rightfully neutral while the other three were supporters of the dispensary. In other words the meeting failed to educate or sway anyone toward our cause. It had been a complete waste of time. If there was a silver lining – looking back on it now I'm not sure there was – we had at least tried. An invitation had been placed in the newspaper asking concerned citizens to attend. You can lead a horse to water…

A week later we were bouncing down the road to Holbrook for yet another Board of Supervisor's Meeting. This, we hoped, would be the meeting to end all meetings. Why would the county deny us the special use permit after contacting us about reopening the discussion? It made absolutely no sense. But then little did in our plight with the county. In addition to the standard showing by Bob, Dusty, and myself we were accompanied by Heather, Jason Scott, and our medical director, Dr. Seth Black.

The meeting commenced with a prayer from a newly elected board member. Isn't there supposed to be a separation of church and state? Not only did she mention Jesus (though she might have been referring to Mormon Jesus) but she also wanted everyone to bow their heads for the Obama administration to guide us through these tough times. Worse yet, she's a republican.

First up on the agenda was a proclamation setting aside a special day known as *Day of the Cougar* in honor of a big state win for the Show Low Junior High (Cougars) wrestling team. Though it was neat and all, I couldn't fathom how winning the state junior high wrestling tournament equated to a special day set aside let alone 45 minutes at a county board meeting. I soon had my answer…One of the supervisor's kids was on the team. Say no more.

After the wrestlers – all twenty-five of them – left the cramped room to head back to school, those of us left standing in their stead, Dusty and I included, were able to finally find a seat. The first item of business was the purchase of a new truck. Apparently the truck was some sort of insurance claim replacement for one that had been stolen. I'm not sure why someone would want to steal a county truck with a huge county emblem on the door but I did once come across a school district car parked out in the woods near my house so I guess it does happen. A bevy of fluoride-treatment grant presentations was followed up by a discussion on how the county was going to be reimbursed by DEA and Homeland Security following recent joint task force operations. Just as I thought we were going to delve into our special use permit hearing a stout fellow in a suit waddled down to the podium with a yawningly shoddy presentation on county budget concerns. As if the material weren't dreary enough the man compounded the dreariness with his own ineptitude often forgetting what it was he wanted to say. I can only hope he is better at crunching numbers than presenting them.

At long last the time had come for our public hearing. To bolster our chances a lawyer named Adam Trenk from the Rose Law Group was on hand to present our case to the board. We met the man for the first time minutes before the meeting. As I said earlier, communication between clients wasn't deemed all that important to the Rose Law Group. Trenk, dashing in an expensive suit and red tie, frequently used the word *power* during his presentation. Though he certainly was eloquent, he didn't present anything that wasn't presented at the prior meetings, he just sounded and looked better than Bob or I did while doing it. Aside from two changes in board membership the only real difference between the prior meeting and the present was a list of concessions (see below) aimed at softening the board's stance.

Overgaard Compassion Care agrees that the Special Use Permit for a Medical Marijuana Dispensary shall be subject to the following stipulations:

- The dispensary shall not conduct business between the hours of 6:30am and 8:00am, or between the hours of 3:00pm and 5:00pm on weekdays, in order to ensure there is no traffic into or out of the dispensary when the Heber-Overgaard School District Busses are running at or near the Facility.

- The dispensary shall not be open past 7:00pm any day of the week.

- The dispensary shall not be open for business on Sundays.

- External signage shall be restricted to two small signs. One double-sided sign no larger than four feet by three feet to be visible to traffic on the road side kiosk/marquee in front of the facility, and one single sided sign no larger than four foot by five foot on the front of the facility. There shall be no other external signage. There will be no outward indication on the signs that the business conducted at the facility is related to marijuana in any way.

136

Green lettering, a green cross, and/or symbols or slang for the word "Marijuana" or its components shall be strictly prohibited.

- The appearance of the building will be maintained to reflect the appearance of medical office space.

- The dispensary operator shall provide all the safety assurances, security and monitoring systems, strict non-loitering enforcement and operate in strict compliance with all security requirements as mandated by Arizona Department of Health Services ("AZDHS"), to ensure public safety.

- No minors, under 18 years of age, will be permitted in the dispensary unless accompanied by a parent or guardian.

- Patron access to the dispensary shall be limited to those individuals possessing an AZDHS issued Patient or Caregiver Identification Card.

- The dispensary operator shall establish a Community Liaison position within its agency, to listen to and address the concerns and issues of the community and collaborate with community leaders as needed. The contact information for the

Community Liaison will be provided to the County Sheriff's office for ease of contact to immediately address any concerns.

- The Special Use Permit shall be subject to a review by the County Board of Supervisors at a public hearing one year from the date the dispensary facility opens for business (following authorization to operate from AZDHS). The Special Use Permit may be revoked at that hearing in the event the Dispensary Operator has violated any of these stipulations, the laws of the State of Arizona, or any local laws or regulations.

Trenk even saw fit to throw in a few concessions that weren't on the original list – a list we had grudgingly consented to. The add-on concessions hadn't been considered let alone agreed upon. Shrugging over in Dusty's direction, I figured all would be forgotten as long as the special use came our way. We'd deal with reality when the need arose. No sooner had Trenk sat down than the drubbing began. Old hat to Dusty, Bob and I, it was a novel experience for Heather, Jason, and Seth.

Heading out from the on-deck circle a stately gentleman pranced to the podium spewing a venomous diatribe condemning the 'utter deterioration of society'. Commencing with 'In 1957 after the Korean War…' – the man went on and on complaining to the board that civilization gone to the dogs and marijuana was surely at the crux of it all. I was hoping to hear the man make mention of Woodstock or the Summer of Love, but it never materialized. He did however mention the fact that casinos had led to society's downfall. I held my snickering to a light murmuring not quite sure where he was going with his line of thought, as three out of five board members were Indians and the only sort of casinos we have in Arizona are Indian casinos. He rambled on about the high price of marijuana then turned to the audience and admitted he had no idea how much the stuff cost, 'but it had to be expensive'. He never came close to making a point concerning the special use permit. In closing he muttered: 'Gosh I think I'd be buying a few seeds and growing them in my yard.'

The Cry Baby (the owner of the adjacent body shop), dressed in his familiar black t-shirt and jacket, brought up the same issues as he had earlier. The only difference being a jab aimed directly at me. He claimed someone (that someone being me) had confronted him at the previous meeting. In reality, it had been the Cry Baby who had invaded my personal space by making barbed comments while we all stood around waiting for the board to render a verdict on the special use permit. I calmly asked whether it seemed safe to have kids running around his body shop with so many dangerous things lying here and there such as wrecked vehicles and machinery. My question set him in a tizzy and before I knew it I could damn near make out what he had had for breakfast.

An old man shuffled up to the dais clutching a handful of yellow, wrinkly papers. If you closed your eyes you might have believed you were listening to Mr. Mackey on the television show *South Park*. Talking in endless circles, Mackey II trotted out a marijuana study from the Vietnam War. Yes, the Vietnam War! Reading from his discolored papers the man listed the hair-raising hazards marijuana had presented G.I.s while fighting in Vietnam. Straight-faced and serious he professed "marijuana had caused a good many soldier to overdose." He failed to mention bullets, land mines, Agent Orange, or even syphilis as factors leading to the deaths of G.I.s.

A woman I'll refer to here as the Camel Lady, as it was she who graced us with the euphemism at the previous BOS meeting, brought a true sense of unintentional humor to the podium. In a voice filled with conviction and moral sagacity, the Camel Lady relayed to the crowd a sordid story she had seen recently on the television news. She explained how Jan Brewer, the governor of Arizona, had recently flown over the Arizona-Mexican border in a 'Black Heart' helicopter and couldn't believe what she saw. According to the Camel Lady, Jan Brewer 'had seen with her own eyes' legions of cartel personnel lining up to invade Arizona dispensaries in what would surely become an international turf war of epic proportion. What do you even say to people like this?

The topic of profit coursed through the meeting as if it had its own pulse. Of course we were hoping to have profits, lots of them in fact. Why else would we put ourselves through all this agony? I wanted to ask the crowd if they believed Pfizer was in business to lose money.

If there was a highlight to the meeting it was the impassioned speech delivered by Heather detailing her own personal bout with breast cancer. Presenting details, she relayed her struggle to form an appetite and shake the effects of chemotherapy. Heather (who is by no means a woman who breaks down easily) tearfully explained the benefits medical marijuana had offered her. The room grew quiet, even the detractors sympathizing for Heather in her plight. As Heather sat down a man jumped up out if his chair and raced to the dais to set the record straight, berating anyone using medical marijuana to ease nausea or pain in any way, shape, or manner. 'It's all just a scam', he maliciously bellowed. 'Don't believe a word of it.' From the very onset the man's tone did more damage than good to his cause. Heather's story had been both sad and sincere no matter what side of the medical marijuana issue one claimed. To publicly attack in such a vicious manner was downright uncivil, embarrassing even to the Camel Lady and the Cry Baby. As the man rambled on pointlessly, Bob, sitting to my left, began convulsing with ire, his neck and head a deep crimson shade. We had agreed in advance that none of the team, spare lawyer Trenk, would speak but Bob had heard enough. No sooner had the man relinquished the dais, Bob had risen to his feet and was walking toward the pulpit. Unleashing a torrent of fury at the man regarding his statements aimed at undermining Heather's credibility, he reiterated what everyone in the room surely had to be thinking, that the man was a cruel, uncaring lump of humanity. I believe Bob would have stormed the dais even had he not known the aggrieved party, fortunately we weren't sitting in a bar or things might have gotten very ugly.

Leaving the meeting I felt ethereal, as if I were floating. The deflating feeling was surreal; we had lost yet again to Boss Hogg and his minions. Worse yet we had been dragged through the mud. As 'the team' gathered for an unappetizing post-meeting meal at a Mexican restaurant in Holbrook, I silently wondered if the food was really as bad as it seemed or whether the bad taste left in my mouth from the meeting made it seem that way. Perhaps a little of both. For all intents and purposes the project seemed doomed. As we made our way back home to Overgaard the energy and fervor I once possessed drained from my soul.

PART III

Reassessment

"You Guys were Mormonized!"

Licking our wounds in the aftermath of the most recent defeat at the hands of the board of supervisors I was told by several people around town that we had basically been 'Mormonized'. They explained that we would never make a go of it in a town run – as Heber and Overgaard surely are – by Mormons. Over the years I've come to know a great deal of Mormons. Come to think of it, it's hard to say anything bad about a single one of them. Most, if not all, have been hard-working, honest people. As a freedom-oriented individual, I don't condemn anyone for believing what they want to believe – no matter how fanatical or fantastical – as long as it doesn't infringe on my own rights. You want to worship the devil…Go for it. You want to pray to the sun…Be my guest. Just don't ask or expect me to buy into your faith-based principles if you truly trust that your holy scripture magically appeared to a man peering lovingly into a white stovepipe hat. I don't mean to sound snide it's just that very little about Mormonism makes much sense to me. For instance, a monumental battle was allegedly fought on a hill in New York with over two million people losing their lives, yet to this day not one shred of evidence has been discovered. No arrowheads. No swords. No bones or mass gravesites. Nothing. Nada. Zip. How can that possibly be? Mormonism was purportedly around for 1400 years prior to Joseph Smith doing his thing with the plates in the hat yet we find nothing in the way of artifactual substance or documentary evidence to support it. No coins. No ruins. No tools. No written history. What's more the place names in the Book of Mormon don't correspond to any modern place names. Not one. Same goes for the hokey maps found in the Book of Mormon. Where are these places anyway? I'll give you a hint…They don't exist. They never did and they never will. If these people sailing across the wide Atlantic really existed, what happened to them all? Neither the Mayans, nor any other indigenous tribe ever mentioned them. The Book of Mormon talks about horses and other beasts of burden. The first horse can be traced only as far back as the arrival of Spanish Conquistadores. Five hundred years ago. There are claims of metalworking and steel. Where was it smelted? There are descriptions of Maya-like structures such as those found at Tikal and Palenque. Where are they? I'm not trying to belittle or demean. I'm just underwhelmed that's all. Had Joseph Smith suffocated during those long, dreamy spells in the hat, we might never have even heard of Mormonism. Here's what one of my heroes Mark Twain had to say about the Book of Mormon in *Roughing It*:

"All men have heard of the Mormon Bible, but few except the 'elect' have seen it, or, at least, taken the trouble to read it. I brought away a copy from Salt Lake. The book is a curiosity to me, it is such a pretentious affair, and yet so 'slow,' so sleepy; such an insipid mess of inspiration. It is chloroform in print. If Joseph Smith composed this book, the act was a miracle — keeping awake while he did it was, at any rate. If he, according to tradition, merely translated it from certain ancient and mysteriously-engraved plates of copper, which he declares he found under a stone, in an out-of-the-way locality, the work of translating was equally a miracle, for the same reason.

"The book seems to be merely a prosy detail of imaginary history, with the Old Testament for a model; followed by a tedious plagiarism of the New Testament. The author labored to give his words and phrases the quaint, old-fashioned sound and structure of our King James's translation of the Scriptures; and the result is a mongrel — half modern glibness, and half ancient simplicity and gravity. The latter is awkward and constrained; the former natural, but grotesque by the contrast. Whenever he found his speech growing too modern — which was about every sentence or two — he ladled in a few such Scriptural phrases as 'exceeding sore,' 'and it came to pass,' etc., and made things satisfactory again. 'And it came to pass' was his pet. If he had left that out, his Bible would have been only a pamphlet."

"It seems a pity he [Smith] did not finish, for after all his dreary former chapters of commonplace, he stopped just as he was in danger of becoming interesting."

"The Mormon Bible is rather stupid and tiresome to read, but there is nothing vicious in its teachings. Its code of morals is unobjectionable --it is "smouched" [Milton] from the New Testament and no credit given."

~

Though there was certainly some degree of truth to what these people were saying – that we had been Mormonized – plenty of other dispensaries in places like downtown Phoenix were also being denied special use permits. I guess what I'm trying to say is this…While Mormons were opposed to the notion of a dispensary in their backyard there were plenty of non-Mormons holding similar views.

Tabla Rasa

Mere days after the coup de grâce had been delivered, the Navajo County Planning and Zoning manager emailed me, informing us that he wanted to help find us a new location, even offering to drive around with us. Whether he was acting on his own volition or someone above him was pulling his strings is anyone's guess. He said he located a piece of property and in doing so it just happened to be the same land mentioned in the BOS meeting. Coincidence? Again, I'm not sure. In the course of the previous meeting a man named Porter had mentioned owning property on the outskirts of Overgaard that met all of our zoning requirements. For some the word outskirts relates to something on the periphery, but in this particular case the word referred to property nearly twelve long miles out of town with virtually nothing in between. Speaking of nothing, other than a rundown sawmill and a gathering pen for range cows, there is absolutely nothing, and I mean nothing, around Porter's piece of property aside from tumbling sagebrush and windswept dirt. To this day I'm still not altogether sure whether Porter ever intended to lease a portion of his land to us. He could well have been speaking in jest at the meeting as if to say: 'Hey, there are a lot of options outside town'.

One thing led to another and before you knew it we were in negotiations. Though Porter owns a 12-acre parcel bordering the sawmill (which he also carries a note on), he was unwilling to lease us anything larger than a half-acre, postage stamp-sized parcel flanked by an unrented billboard and a 400-foot cell tower. Furthermore, he was wholly unwilling to sell us the land…At any price it seemed. Incongruously enough, cell phone reception is terrible at the site.

All the grousing we had done concerning the installation of a HVAC system in the shopping plaza in Overgaard suddenly seemed trite to the point of banal. Everything had been set and ready to go at the small shopping plaza in town and here we were faced with the challenge of starting anew in a dirt field lacking even one utility source – for there was no water or electricity – forced to slap together a half-assed temporary set-up in the span of several months. Worse yet, we were forced to remodel over our remodeling efforts prior to handing the suites in the shopping center back to the landlord. Talk about a depressing chore.

Springtime is a windy period in the mountains of the Southwest. With few large trees to impede flow, the new location reminded me of Rawlins, Wyoming – desolate and windswept. A minute or two out there and you found yourself covered head to toe in fine red dust. Faced with the decision of folding up the tents and moving on to unknown endeavors (we had no viable backup plan) or 'taking our medicine' and making a go of it on Porter's land, we capitulated, abruptly whisked into a world of building inspectors and tradesmen.

First there was the state highway department to deal with as an 'egress' had to be figured out. Egress was nothing more than an extravagant way of saying we needed a driveway with an approach apron after hacking our way through a state fence designed to keep cows from wandering out onto the highway. Fortunately Bob Fern became chummy with the head man at the Arizona Department of Transportation (ADOT) office in Show Low and he agreed to allow entry to the property via what he referred to as temporary range access status. The assigned status meant we could temporarily avoid constructing a more permanent asphalt driveway and apron which could have easily cost more than $15,000. The range access status on the other hand allowed us to pile up dirt and rocks over the ditch beside the highway. After cutting the state fence to access the site we had to install a tubular ranch gate on the property. Knowing absolutely nothing about such things Dusty and I made our way to Show Low where we purchased a 14' gate because a 12' gate was only $5 cheaper. In hindsight we would have been in serious trouble as the doublewide trailer we later purchased would not have cleared the 12' gate opening.

Unable to build something permanent, we embarked on a quest to find something portable yet serviceable. While anything from circus tents to cargo containers were discussed we knew our only real option was some sort of mobile home. Visiting a showroom in Show Low we discovered, to our consternation that new singlewide mobiles were fetching nearly fifty thousand dollars! Stripped singlewide models in Phoenix could be had for around $30,000, but this was much more than we wanted to spend so we sought out used models large and small. No matter the size, one thing remained constant…They all smelled atrocious. Suffering from an acute aversion to mold and mildew, merely entering one of these structures caused me to feel ill for the remainder of the day and sometimes part of the next as well. What does a moldy thirty year-old singlewide go for you ask? According to Leapin' Larry, a man who refurbishes the exhausted structures in Springerville, the answer is $12,000. Twelve thousand smackeroos for a malodorous and beat trailer! Funny thing is that's about what they're worth. Perhaps a little less if you find the right deal but they sure as hell aren't going for two or three thousand dollars as we had previously and erroneously assumed. Add to it the $4,000 dollars (or more) to move and set one of these things and you're talking a real chunk of change.

In the end a decision was made to rent a construction trailer from Mobile Mini. Taking a trip down to Phoenix to investigate what one of these things looked like we were escorted across the highway by a salesman on a Harley who showed us around a metropolis of units big and small, every last one of them white in color. Aside from the $4,000 delivery and set up fee a one-year lease seemed highly affordable at only $250 a month. Or it was until walking back through the dusty parking lot the sales agent mentioned quite casually that it was another $250 a month to rent the handicapped ramp to access the trailer. We wondered how this could possibly be. A steel ramp cost as much to rent as an entire trailer? I suppose they're going get you one way or another…

Just as the trailer was to be delivered the agent from Mobile Mini called to ensure we had obtained the requisite permit required to set the trailer on the lot. Dusty, talking to the man on his cell phone looked over at me with inquisitive eyes as if I might have had any more insight into the matter than he did. I didn't. We hadn't filed any paperwork for the permit because we hadn't known a permit had been required. It wasn't the first nor the last time we were to learn the hard way when it came to governmental officialdom.

After ironing out the permit snafu the trailer arrived in a howling wind several days later. Due to what had been described as a 'bad axle' the driver delivering the trailer had gone through five spare tires on the trip up from Phoenix. The driver's harrowing assessment simply begged the question. 'How many spare tires did you have with you?' Glancing over at me with a sheepish grin the driver humbly replied: 'Five'. We had solved one part of the puzzle. We now had ourselves a dispensary storefront. At 12' wide and 44' long it would surely be the tiniest storefront in the state, but we didn't fret, it was a start.

~

Storefront issue solved we concentrated on the next problem…What were we going to do about a grow facility? Without a grow facility the entire venture would be sunk. While it's possible to make a few bucks selling other people's product the real money lay in growing your own. I once used a pizza analogy when explaining our situation to Trent Larson down at planning and zoning. "I have a pizza business but no ovens or any means of producing pizzas. I buy pizzas from next door for $6 and sell them for $8. That's not bad right, but think how many pizzas you would have to sell to make a profit let alone pay your overhead and employees." I'm not sure he got the analogy or perhaps he didn't care, but that's about the gist of it when it comes to medical marijuana.

Our first thought was to grow outdoors. With the growing season fast approaching a good many plants could be grown on a quarter acre of open land. I began researching *hoopdees*, those plasticky greenhouse-like contraptions you see on marijuana programs. Five hundred dollars (labor not included) bought you a half-decent setup. Full-sized greenhouses were another option or were until ADHS (the state overseer for medical marijuana) informed us each greenhouse (including hoopdees) would require a toilet and a sink. Furthermore, any outdoor grow required a ten-foot high fence around it. Not chain link mind you, a solid fence constructed out of concrete, metal, or stone. Crack math told us a fence of that nature would cost around $100 a square foot! $60,000-$80,000 dollars. Even if one was inclined to shell out the cash, there was no guarantee the fence could withstand the high winds sweeping across the desolate plains. Besides, a ten-foot high fence creates a great deal of shade thereby rendering much of the fence's perimeter wholly unsuitable for cultivation.

The more we thought about things, the more the outdoor grow idea appeared doomed. It would have been one thing had we owned the land. But constructing a high-dollar fence with concrete footings which would have to be removed when we left the property was absurd. Switching gears, we began running the numbers on cargo containers. Without a long term lease or a deed to the land it just didn't make any sense to build anything permanent. Cargo containers certainly weren't ideal. Hot in the summer, cold in the winter, they lacked both space and efficiency. Joking that we had always discussed acquiring cargo containers for one reason or another, Dusty and I visited a local retailer in Linden. Escorted around the back lot by a couple of people certainly looking the part of cargo container salespeople, we discussed the options of installing doors and windows. They said it would take several weeks to have one delivered and that was before any torching was completed. Showing me the calendar on the wall I couldn't fathom the number of people purchasing used cargo containers. Preppers I suppose. We said we'd have to think about it.

A few days later we received a 'hot tip' on a trio of cargo containers located north of Phoenix at a friend of a friend's compound. Dusty and I set out to investigate. Originally intending to bury the containers in the ground, the doors had been removed from two of the containers. These open ends were then intended to (I say intended to because they never actually were physically connected) connect to the broad side of the third container forming what appeared to me to be a subterranean space station of sorts. Before the project got off the ground the neighbors complained about the abundant noise and dust and the project came to a complete halt. After a change in plans the trio of cargo containers had become obsolete and available to someone in the market for such an arrangement. After examining the setup we pretty much gave up on the idea of a cargo container grow facility. Limited by the amount of usable space and plagued by large temperature swings, we felt there had to be a better option available. As to what that better option was we weren't quite certain so we went back to focusing on the storefront as it was absolutely essential in obtaining the licensure and special use permit from the county.

Planning on using a gray water system for our sinks and a black water system for our toilet we began gathering information to that end only to be instructed by the county that a septic tank would be required. Two days later an "engineer" named Bob and a backhoe operator named Lee showed up to dig test holes for the percolation test. Following Bob the engineer around for much of the morning I learned a great deal more than I ever cared to know about perc tests and soil composition. Happy with what they found, a concrete tank was dropped in place several days later.

Septic in place, we still had no water. Our options were few. Bring in a large holding tank and have water delivered or run lines from an existing well located over a quarter mile away. Neither option was cheap but the hassle of dealing with the sawmill people for water persuaded us to purchase a tank and rely on deliveries from a water-hauling woman from nearby Clay Springs.

In addition to our dearth of water, we also lacked electricity leading directly to the property. On a visit to the local electricity company, a beleaguered woman behind an exceedingly unorganized desk assured us it was no big deal. A day or two later the story changed. Informed we needed a commercial bypass requiring expensive equipment and a long lag time for parts, the electrical job suddenly went from quick fix to lengthy ordeal. Our backhoe man Lee recommended a local electrician named Keith for the job. Accompanied by his nephew Winston (the name reminding me of Orwell's main character in *1984*), Keith met us out at the site to sort out our options. As a Mormon, Keith was naturally opposed to medical marijuana, but told me 'as long as it's legal then I'm okay with it. 'Tobacco and alcohol, I might not approve of these things but they're legal. 'An abortion clinic on the other hand…No way, in fact I'd pull the wiring out before I installed any. 'Better yet I'd reverse the polarity!' I had heard this theory from Mormons before. It didn't make much sense then and it didn't now. We're discussing legality here not morality. Abortion clinics are just as legal as liquor stores or smoke shops under Arizona law. I began to explain this to Keith and then bit my tongue knowing my explanation would never sink in.

A week later he mentioned the same story about sabotaging the abortion clinic. Listening for a short time I changed the subject. As I changed the subject Lee the backhoe man asked Keith whether or not he enjoyed an occasional Mountain Dew. 'All the time', replied both Keith and Winston simultaneously. Those rebellious Mormons. Shunning alcohol and tobacco, caffeine is also considered a no-no, although a light one. Mountain Dew is the overwhelming choice in soft drinks for Mormons, so much so that it's a running joke among Mormons and non-Mormons. Like I always say if you're going to sin you may as well sin big by going with the king of caffeine-laden soda pops.

Lee went on to needle Keith about the Mormon connection to the Pepsi Corporation. 'You know your church owns the damned thing', grinned Lee. 'Oh that's only a myth Lee', cried Keith. After disputing the matter in a joking manner for several minutes Keith explained that back in the 1970s an apostle of the Mormon Church had owned serious shares in the company. The church hierarchy, frowning on such activities forced this apostle to sell his shares. End of the story according to Keith. Lee didn't buy it, saying the church was somehow involved. I just stood by and laughed. First of all, this business about owning Pepsi (others say it is Coca Cola that the Mormons own) is purely bunk. A rumor gone viral. Think of the irony, a religious group admonishing caffeine beverages owning Pepsi. While the church has official doctrine reproaching the use of coffee, tea, tobacco, and alcohol, it only advises its flock to avoid caffeinated beverages such as Mountain Dew. A sugary loophole if you will. As for the rumor end of it, consider Coca Cola, where owning a mere 1% of the corporation would set back an investor over three billion dollars. Before leaving, Keith wished us well and hoped our trailer wouldn't get shot up. Not by ordinary thugs, he chuckled, but by pious Mormons angered by our presence. I simply smiled and thought to myself: What if a Mormon temple got shot up? After all, plenty of people don't care for Mormonism any more than they care for marijuana.

About Schmitt

When it appeared Porter was completely intent on *not* selling us any of his land, I decided other options were necessary. Driving down Highway 277 between Snowflake and Overgaard, I had often espied green and white *Forest Properties* signs. Ironically, though I'd seen these realty signs sticking out of the ground beside all manner of highway and byway, I'd never once seen one on property with any real tree cover, let alone something resembling a forest. *Scrub Properties* is surely a more apt name. From what I gleaned, the company seemed to own or broker the only property for sale in either direction for ten miles, maybe further. After doing a little research on the company I shot an email to a man named Don Schmitt through his Forest Properties website explaining what we wanted: 4-5 acres of power-ready highway frontage zoned commercial or industrial. A few days later I received a return email informing me he had exactly what we were looking for. Tersely informing me he was averse to using email as a form of communication, Don wrote that it would be better to contact him by phone. Heeding his instructions I called the man up for a chat. I soon wished I hadn't. From the very onset Don didn't come across as someone trying to sell land. Combative and argumentative, he told me on no less than six occasions he had 'a background in law'. What that meant I still haven't a clue. I was forced to take four or five stats classes in college, but for the life of me, I wouldn't begin informing people that I had a background in statistics. Besides, if you are selling something, anything for that matter, does it not behoove you to be amenable or at the very least rational? Why on earth would you be argumentative when talking on the phone to someone who may be interested in purchasing your land? Remember this was land in the middle of nowhere. Suspect scrub land on a windswept plain.

After ranting and raving like a lunatic – I really began thinking the man was stoned drunk – Don finally calmed down long enough for me to explain in further detail what we were looking for. 'Well… what do you have in mind for this land', he bellowed into the phone. A facility in the form of a large metal structure or pole barn, I explained. 'What???' 'I have deed restrictions and I don't want to see any junk around.' Taken aback, I almost fell off the chair I was leaning back in. I replied very cordially that I didn't say anything about junk; that I was referring to an aesthetically pleasing compound of tastefully built structures constructed from the finest of modern materials. 'There's already a lot of junk around here I don't think we can do any business at this time!' Hanging up the phone I was rather in shock. I didn't quite know what to make of the quirky conversation. Don had land and we needed land. I called Dusty and told him someone else would have to line up as cannon fodder. I thought Bob Fern, a man who thoroughly enjoys talking to people on the phone was perfect for the job but for some reason he refused to make the call. We decided to engage a realtor we had known for some time, but she too seemed hesitant to call the man. The more people we talked to the more legendary Don's reputation grew. 'Oh that guy, yeah I know him, deal with his son if you can…' A stroke was mentioned which seemed to explain the ranting behavior I took for drunkenness, but then I wasn't so sure.

Though my conversation with Don went horribly wrong I still wasn't ready to give up. For one thing there just wasn't any land to be had (talking with Porter again regarding his land, he gave the impression he was adamant about not selling 'at this time') and secondly, I thought if the man sounded like that on the phone, just think what he'd be like in person. If nothing else it would be entertaining.

Wanting to avoid tipping our hand with another phone conversation, Dusty and I decided a pop-in visit to Don's office was the best plan of action. Driving the 36 odd miles over to Snowflake, Dusty and I found Don sitting behind a cluttered desk, easy listening music blaring from a nearby radio. To say Don resembled a cartoon character would be completely underestimating the visualization. The self-proclaimed 82 year-old broker immediately began berating us the moment we walked in the door. Partially concealed behind bushy eyebrows, and a prodigious schnozz protruding bridge hairs, Don reminded me for the seventh time that he had a background in law. Not only that, but he knew a thing or two about the medical field as well. And insurance and banking, 'hell, he'd been in the business for over 50 years'. After each and every sentence he uttered: 'Anyway, all's I'm saying is...' If I would have had a meter on it, I'm sure it would have registered in the hundreds. As he grumbled on about this or that I began feeling sort of sorry for the guy. I found myself thinking: I sure hope I never act like this.

I assure you, even now in the twilight of his life, Don's not the kind of man you can bull over. He's the type of person in which you strap tap shoes on your feet before entering his office. Or for that matter talking to him on the telephone. Don spoke of past events as if they had happened just yesterday although in reality they occurred some forty years earlier. Handing a couple letters of recommendation from 1988 (the year I graduated from college) for my perusal, Don dropped the names of long-forgotten senators and judges we might have known. He spoke of soirées and cocktail parties, hobnobbing with power families of vintage Arizona. As a historian, I found it amusing to listen to his nostalgic tales. How much of what he was saying was true, I can only speculate. He spoke of lawyers and insurance and banking and business. He said he built up the business with only 5,000 dollars in the 1960s. Come to think of it, Don spoke of nearly everything but the price of his 12-acre parcel in the outback.

After finally pinning him down by asking to see a map of the area, he went into a lengthy discourse involving the social stigma of marijuana and how he didn't want it to devalue his other holdings in the area. At times it sounded as if he was ready to deal, and then reluctance clouded his thoughts. Don said the land would eventually fall into the hands of his son, so it might be wise to consult him. Later, when I revisited the topic by saying perhaps we should talk to his son about the project, he looked me straight in the eye with a crazed look before blurting out 'it's my land damnit, you don't look a gift horse in the mouth do you?'

Don, mentioning for the tenth time that he had a background in law was eager to know if we had a lawyer. It then took ten minutes for him to write down the lawyer's name and his law firm. Each time he'd write the name down he'd search around aimlessly for a paper clip or a stapler and feeling useless, I wanted to pass these items to him but knew better. He had once inquired what happened to the business card Dusty had handed him and I told him that he had placed in the drawer. 'What?' 'No, I would never do that!' A minute or two later Don located the card – in the drawer. For some reason he wanted to ensure us the zoning would work even if he was yet unwilling to actually deal us the land. He looked in the phone book and fumbled around with the phone trying to raise someone at planning and zoning in Holbrook. Thankfully no one was there to talk to him. As he reread Dusty's name on the business card he suddenly barked out the name 'Dusty Parsons', imploring if we were familiar with the man. We said no and then he began dialing up the planning and zoning number once more. When the secretary answered he asked if Dusty Parsons was the former planning and zoning director. The secretary, not sure why he was asking, became befuddled. Don amped up by annoyance posed the same question (only louder) a few more times until the secretary simply agreed with him. Banging down the receiver, Don looked at us with a twinkle in his cataract-plagued eyes exclaiming 'see there, always good to have a name to drop when you talk to these people.' My head nodded but my stomach roiled.

Vacillating back and forth, Don went from offering his expertise to our business plan to adamantly proclaiming he wasn't interested in what we had to say. During an upswing Don urged us to attain real estate licenses so we could make a few bucks selling his land.

"All it takes is a few hours on the idiot box [pointing to a computer] to acquire a license', he roared. He then mentioned visiting a mobile home dealer down the road to acquire something tasteful so the value of his adjacent holdings wouldn't be diminished. By the time we got up to leave we didn't know what to think. As we walked to the door Don asked if we were interested in some coffee. We thanked him but said no. As for the music, it was still blaring; Don had never thought to turn it down.

~

Several visits and phone calls followed with similar results. In other words, very little progress toward any tangible result was realized. Months later, after Heather had arrived from Ohio, we drove out so that she could meet Don. It was readily apparent Don was a lady's man by the way his personality softened in the presence of a woman. What didn't change however was Don's shrewd business etiquette. When I reminded Don what he had quoted us as a price on the land several months earlier he immediately balked, looking over at me through those bushy eyebrows of his as if I were insane, counter-offering with a price nearly twice as high. Through all of Don's idiosyncrasies I really began taking a fondness for the man. Unfortunately, fondness only gets you so far.

Three's a Charm...BOS III

After all the drama of the previous meetings, both comedic and tragic, the planning and zoning and board of supervisor's hearings concerning our new location turned out to be snoring non-events. Whereas at the earlier meetings hostile mobs had packed the room in oppositional solidarity, the room now fell eerily silent, not one person attending to voice antipathy toward our new project. This is what the county desired. They didn't want to go on record as rigid, uncaring ogres slamming the door on medical marijuana patients. On the other hand they didn't want to appear chummy with the likes of dispensary owners by allowing the most sensible option – a dispensary in town. The message was clear: If you take your weed business out to the hinterlands – where we can't see it – then we'll grant you the special use permit. And so they did.

Board members outnumbered attendees as Dusty, his friend Lee from Ohio, and I were the only souls in attendance at the planning and zoning meeting. It had been so long since we had faced the planning and zoning board (six months) I wasn't sure whether they were the same members or not. I was assured by Homero Vela from planning and zoning that they were but I still wasn't so sure. After a summary by Homero, I offered to answer questions from the board. One of the male board members desired posing a question specifically to Dusty. Dusty, standing at the dais stated that he would rather have me answer the question.

Brows furrowed, the board member commented that for someone claiming to own a, Dusty sure did come off as vague and uncooperative. Dusty, bristling momentarily, explained he was well aware of everything going on with the dispensary but it wasn't his strong suit to speak about it. Dusty's reply ended the board member's proddings and after several more questions the board put the motion to a vote which was nearly unanimous aside from a tele-attending board member on speaker phone who might actually have intended to vote in favor but abstained in the midst of what sounded like burping.

~

Five days later we were back in Holbrook for the board of supervisor's meeting. Though a small throng had assembled, none of them were there for us – or shall I say there to oppose us – all being there for other reasons. Following several curious prayers we sat through a long list if business not pertaining to our cause. There was a proposed wind turbine survey project adjacent to Farmer John's pig farm. No, I didn't make that up. Not once did anyone mention Farmer John's last name, only referring to the farm and or the farmer as Farmer John. The project's head honcho, jetting in from the state of Washington, explained that he needed to erect a tower or two in order to make sure there was enough wind in the area to make the project viable. Granted approval, he was given two years to do the testing, after which the towers would have to be dismantled and removed.

Several cases before the board involved residents disputing tax assessments on their mobile homes.

While I certainly consider any attempt to battle the forces of government noble, these particular cases made little sense. Had these citizens won their appeals – they didn't – the tax savings could only have amounted to marginal savings. The mobiles were being taxed at a value of $15,000. Had they been able to whittle that figure down to let's say $13,500 they might have hoped to save perhaps $10 on their taxes. It cost more than that in gas to drive to Holbrook from Show Low.

When a proposed storage facility came up for discussion Dusty and I glanced over at each other with nodding smirks, knowing it was a done deal when an engineer with a prominent Mormon name stepped to the podium to explain the ins and outs of the project. A concerned neighbor explained that his house was directly behind the proposed facility, stressing the point that his bedroom window would be flooded by the proposed lighting of the facility. 'Besides there are already two storage facilities in the area that aren't full, so why do we need another one?' It was a valid point, but the man, who in his heart perhaps realized it, had no chance. Whisked away, he retreated to his chair where he witnessed a unanimous vote in favor of the storage facility. On a more humorous note there had been an email complaint by the state of Arizona, which owned a large tract of undeveloped land just to the east of the proposed facility. The state was apparently concerned about dust issues. As one of the board members read the complaint laughter erupted from not only the audience but the board itself. Here was a dust-inducing, desolate tract of state land and THEY were worried about dust? I decided it had to be a joke. I hope anyway.

Our hearing came last. Without a shred of fanfare or controversy the board granted us our long-awaited special use permit. We heard several days later that two of the board members had mentioned, after the meeting had already concluded, that they would have preferred to have voted against our special use permit. But as the vote had already been tallied it was more of a publicity stunt than anything else. We had the county's blessing. We had prevailed, though it was a hollow victory with little fanfare or enthusiasm. Instead of a shopping center full of opportunity we had been exiled to Siberia.

Finger Lickin' Cashew Chicken

While being a licensed drug dealer may sound glamorous to some, I can assure there was no end to the tedious chores confronting us on an everyday basis and we hadn't even sold our first gram. And Unlike ordinary everyday drug dealers we failed to possess lackeys to do our dirty work. This meant we were obligated to learn about things we never in our lives wanted to consider. How many tons of 'dirty cinders' were necessary to fill out a pad for a mobile home? How many gallons did you say that water tank held? What was the make again on that unsightly mobile? Is a permit required to move a mobile? Better yet, what doesn't require a permit? Every time we turned around we were acquiring another permit for something. Does the place have to be handicap accessible? The nuances between 200 and 400 amp service panels. The maddening lag time involved with everything...'That'll be two to three weeks...'

~

One morning Dusty and I headed down the mountain to Phoenix to run errands. It's a six-hour minimum roundtrip so it's imperative to kill two or three birds with one stone if possible. Leaving home at 8 o'clock in the morning we arrived in Payson at nine. I needed to have two sets of fingerprints taken for my agent card (a $500 card necessary to work or volunteer in an Arizona dispensary). The address didn't jump out at us so we continued on down the road, thinking we'd do a better job of finding the place in the afternoon on the return journey. Foremost on our mission's to do list was the acquisition of a surveillance system for the dispensary. We also needed to pick up a five-foot glass display cabinet but still hadn't heard back from the company constructing it in Phoenix. Low and behold they phoned as we sped past the charming hamlet of Rye, located ten miles below Payson. Things were coming together. The fewer trips to Phoenix the better, especially now that the scorching heat of summer was right around the corner.

Picking up the cabinet from a factory on West Van Buren Street (the prostitutes linger further east); we jumped back on the crowded freeway and headed for an address I had jotted down from the internet. According to the website the place sold everything we needed: Cameras, monitors, backup batteries, DVRs... However, upon pulling into the parking lot we weren't quite sure what, if anything, the place vended. Sleepwalking through an unmarked door I assumed I had somehow copied down the wrong address. Confused by the outward appearance of the place – boxes of junk stacked here and there – I asked a young woman that just happened to be walking past if we were in the right place. 'Yeah what do you need?' 'Surveillance equipment', I replied still a bit puzzled. 'Oh, okay, I'll see if I can find someone to help you.' Standing there I felt like we had walked in on some sort of front operation for Al Queda or Unitarian Universalism. There were no obvious signs indicating that the place was any sort of business let alone a security business. Several minutes later an Asian

American male, possibly of Korean descent came around the corner and we explained what we needed. Though the website appeared to be a retail storefront the man said he didn't have anything on hand but 'could order what we needed'. How much for a system meeting our needs, we inquired? 'Oh, I'd say around $5,500 for the equipment and then of course the install...' I had already priced a system online for around $1,000; I merely wanted to understand the ins and outs before buying it was all. Inwardly shocked we shook his hand and said we'd get back to him. Upon leaving, I swear I saw a suspicious figure flash around the corner but maybe I was just seeing things.

Famished, we stopped for lunch at a Chinese joint in Dusty's old Tempe neighborhood. Here the state was mandating that we had a sink separate from the bathroom in our minuscule 12' x 44' construction trailer but this Chinese, sit-down style restaurant had no restroom. How could this be? Dusty offhandedly remarked: 'Yeah last time I was here I walked around the side of the Laundromat...' I told him that would leave me relieved but wouldn't do much for my dirty hands. Is it me, or does every Chinese restaurant in America have a look and feel of foreignness? I've traveled all over the world and eating in a Chinese restaurant in America makes me feel as if I've been unwittingly transported somewhere else.

After lunch we stopped off at a nearby Best Buy. They had one system in stock but it was inadequate for our needs. Fortunately the cabinet had come in or the trip would have been a total bust.

On the way home we managed to locate the Payson Police Station. We obviously hadn't looked too hard on the way through in the morning and soon discovered we were to pay dearly for our indiscretion. Approaching the window a kindly elderly woman wearing a volunteer badge explained that fingerprinting was only done in the morning. It was now early afternoon. Pleading with her, we asked if we could do it ourselves as the ink and forms were sitting right by the door. 'No, no, I'm afraid that isn't possible.' We explained that we lived an hour away and didn't have such facilities where we came from, was there any way to call someone? She called dispatch but they told her every available cop was busy. Smiling thoughtfully, she said, 'maybe you should find a hotel for the night.' The woman's line of reasoning was ludicrous as we lived an hour away and it was only 1 pm. Exiting the parking lot we passed by several of Payson's finest visiting, I mean patrolling, near their squad cars.

Unwilling to admit defeat we drove down the road to the Gila County Sheriff's office. A hive of activity, law enforcement personnel of every type – sheriff's deputies, Payson Police officers, Department of Public Safety officers (state police) – traipsed in and out of the building as if they were lost. Just as we approached the window a man in hand cuffs lacking a shirt and shoes was hauled past us. Advancing to a counter protected by bullet-proof glass I explained my need for fingerprinting to a crotchety woman with a scowl. 'Not just anyone can ask for fingerprints, you have to have a reason.' As if I would have been there requesting fingerprints just for the hell of it. Instead of pointing this out I explained in my sweetest voice that the state required my fingerprints. They didn't care where or how I obtained them but they wouldn't issue an agent card without them. No, they hadn't sent me anything in writing. No, they didn't mail me any fingerprint cards.

'I'm afraid we can't do it without some kind of order.' Digging even deeper for an even sweeter voice, I plead with the woman to ask someone else if they could offer any insight into the situation. Just as I thought she was going to chastise me she abruptly left the room to speak with someone behind the wall. I imagined several people, feet up on desks, lounging behind the wall. 'Just wait here the Lieutenant will check on it when he gets the time.' Dusty asked how long it would be and was told, with a smirk and a gesture of empty palms, 'it all depends'. Sitting back down on the hard wooden bench, Dusty and I waited. And waited some more, nothing to do but watch cops come and go through an eight-foot passage leading into the bowels of the station. Each and every time someone came through (this was constant mind you) they had to enter a code on the door by pushing a set of metal buttons. By the fourth or fifth entrance we knew the code but then who in their right mind would break into a police station?

Thirty minutes later an officer came through the door with a copy of the medical marijuana regulations. He had never fingerprinted anyone for the program yet but assured me it could be done. Grateful, I thanked him for 'investigating' the situation. There was a catch however. The fingerprinting was done in the booking room and the booking room was backed up with what he described as 'bad boys' at the moment. I was waiting for the music from the television show to cue up. Could we come back in an hour? Without much of a choice (I needed the card) we said we'd be back.

Walking across the street we visited a grow shop dealing in all things necessary for growing top shelf vegetables: Lighting, soils, chemical additives…Of course no one, aside from marijuana cultivators, would lay out large sums on such items. It's comparable to head shops selling bongs and pipes festooned with those puerile stickers proclaiming *for tobacco use only*. The owners of the grow shop, like us, had won the lottery and had been awarded a dispensary license. Having already called for their inspection, they were set to open in a month's time if all went well.

Squandering away a good portion of an hour shooting the breeze, we returned to the sheriff's office where we handed over $15 for the fingerprints and sat back down on the same hard wooden bench. We waited, then waited some more. Finally, after twenty minutes or so, we were instructed to wait outside on yet another hard bench. It was obvious they didn't want anyone to feel comfortable. A K-9 truck, which had been idling in the parking lot since we initially arrived hours earlier, was still idling away. I suppose this was to keep the dog in the back cool but I found it hard to fathom a better system didn't exist. Two other men milled around outside near the hard bench. One said the court had ordered him to obtain a mug shot and fingerprints for some undisclosed reason. Smiling and seemingly carefree, the lanky thirty-something said he was waiting for the revolution to come and then he wouldn't have to waste his time with such trivial matters. To be honest, he didn't look like someone with a busy schedule to maintain. We told him the Payson dispensary would soon open and that seemed to perk him up. The other guy, in his late twenties, was swearing at an old-fashioned contraption – a payphone – while pacing around in circles. He said he was there to 'put in his 24'. Apparently four o'clock in the afternoon was his pre-scheduled time of arrival. It wasn't his first time either. 'Ahh man, you'd think I'd learn.' I made no comment. He seemed to know all the ins and outs of serving a day in county confinement. Inquisitive, I pumped him for information for which he happily offered. Was it communal? Yes. How many in the room? Up to twelve with only one toilet and no privacy when using it. Did it smell? Horribly. He said he normally takes sleeping pills so it makes the time go by faster. Unfortunately, the previous time – I wasn't sure how many times he'd actually done this sort of thing – he'd taken a sleeping pill and because he was a short-time 24-hour man, they made him a trustee and handed him a mop. Half-conscious he sluggishly mopped up and down the corridors. 'This time I only popped half a tab just in case." How's the food, I asked? 'Oh man, it's shit, fuckin' terrible. I spent six months in Globe (the county seat) but at least the food is better there. Here, hah, man it's real bad, green hotdogs and shit. Green! Whatever gets old in Globe they ship up here…'

In the midst of my impromptu interview the lieutenant that so kindly assisted me past the ogre at the window stopped by for a chat on his way to the parking lot. We asked him what he thought about medical marijuana and like most other cops I'd spoken to, he thought the country was headed toward legalization sometime in the near future. He spoke of fighting in Vietnam and smoking Thai stick. He said hard liquor had had a more serious effect on him. A bad experience led him to swear it off completely until very recently. He was now in his late 60s. Shaking hands and wishing us luck in our green venture he made his way to the parking lot. Moments later I was summoned to the booking room.

Once inside the small, disorderly room I was ordered to sit down on yet another hard bench. Though I was there for fingerprints, I felt no different than any of the other criminals passing through the door. That is, the attending policeman, like most policemen, didn't seem capable of turning on or off his robotic booking instincts, treating me like any other entering his domain. Commanded to stand behind a certain tile line on the floor I was told to extend my arms out toward a computerized glass fingerprinting apparatus. Spraying some sort of fluid on my hands the officer grabbed my hand and brought it toward the glass tray. 'Relax your arm he bellowed.' Had I been taller, or my arms longer, this would have been a reasonable request. But as it was my arm was stiff because it was extended beyond its capability of reach. If I had been allowed to move forward six inches everything would have been fine but keeping with the man's rigid protocol – one size fits all keep your toes behind the damned line – I was forced to stretch and of course had absolutely no chance of "relaxing" my arm. Somehow I made it through without hyperextending both elbows and while putting the prints up on the screen the officer muttered the first non-robotic sentence since I entered the room by quipping 'man you have some horrible fingerprints, just terrible.' Confused, I asked why? 'You been working with paper?' Umm, in what way? 'You know paperwork, office stuff.' Well, I'm a writer and I read a lot of books so I suppose that qualifies as working with paper. He went on to explain that people who work in offices often possess worse fingerprints than construction workers or seamen. Apparently the chemicals in paper destroy fingerprints. Intending to make a wisecrack regarding white collar crime, I held my tongue. 'Hell, I don't know if these prints are good enough but if they aren't come back and we'll do it again.' I thought to myself, sure thing, who in their right mind wouldn't want to hang around another four hours down at the sheriff's station in Payson, you never know who you might meet.

Out at "The Windy Joint"

*O*ne afternoon I found myself sitting down at my parent's kitchen table complaining about the wind down at the new dispensary location. I explained that while it was often blustery in town during the spring months the wind out there is over the top ridiculous. Ranting on, I said that the word wind should have been included somewhere in the company name. My mom suddenly exclaimed: 'Why not call it The Windy Joint?' I nearly fell off my chair. This coming from someone so far removed from the marijuana industry it isn't even funny. I treasured the double-meaning behind the name. Pun-ful and witty, the moniker hit the nail right on the head. Unfortunately we're stuck with the name Overgaard Compassion Care even though *the joint* is located 12 miles out of town.

~

A full-sized, double-sided billboard looms no more than three feet from our allotted property line. Prior to dropping the mobile structures on the lot it was the only object serving as shade. The county had bamboozled us into discreet signage by retaining decrees intended for secreting the disapproved location in town. Dusty figured since the billboard was three feet off the property line it would be fair game for a huge sign. Commenting that this would only invite trouble I offered up an alternative...Pay for a nondenominational sign with the slogan: *Feeling achy? Why not reach for a spliff...Medical Marijuana, it's there for you when you need it*...What do you think? Yeah, I know, a little over the top.

On a more serious note, the day that I uttered these silly words marked the first day that I actually conceived of the dispensary as such. As an operating entity. That isn't to say I had doubts as to whether we would open the doors, it's just that that particular day, May 22, 2013, stirred in me a feeling of positivity. Though Dusty and I had spent plenty of time been out at the new location by that time, there seemed to be something magical about installing the alarm and camera surveillance system inside the construction trailer that somehow triggered a transformation in my emotional point of view. To this day I can't explain why, but it really did.

Driving the 11.6 miles from town to the new dispensary location, you just never knew what you might come across. Antelope. Deer. Elk. In the span of a week I'd come across five or six snakes on the highway, most of them squashed. This is fairly commonplace in the desert down south but rare up here in the mountains. They were obviously trying to warm their bodies on the comparatively warmer asphalt. Unfortunately, they failed to incorporate motor vehicles into the equation. Dusty pondered whether it was nature's way of tidying up the gene pool. I didn't think it would impact the gene pool one way or another but then I never claimed to be a biologist. Several years back we noticed it had been a boom year for migratory bats, so why not snakes this time around? I'll never forget riding ATVs in the desert near phoenix years ago when under a full moon the ground crawled with tarantulas. Everywhere you looked tarantulas marched onward toward points unknown. It was the first and only time I witnessed such a spectacle.

But then it's often the animals you least expect to see that throw you for the biggest loops. Take for instance the four chickens foraging near the highway. It was obvious that they were recently abandoned, most likely that very morning as they seemed to remain in the immediate area where they were given the boot. While the act was irresponsible it was also puzzling as the spot where the chickens were milling around was literally out in the middle of nowhere, miles from any town in either direction. If you were going to execute a death sentence why wouldn't you simply butcher the hens up and eat them? With a number of farms and ranches in the area, abandoning chickens in the middle of nowhere goes totally against the grain. Farmers aren't wasters (of anything) and chickens are normally eaten at the sunset of their egg-laying glory days. I concluded it must have been the actions of chicken owners run amok. Weary of the chickens and too spineless to butcher them, they figured they'd just let them loose to fend for themselves. That way, in their mind anyway, the chickens would live on in indefinitely. They perhaps imagined they were being humane in doing so. Unfortunately, feral hens aren't like feral pigs. They can't defend themselves against, well, against really anything that might want to eat them…Coyotes, skunks, raccoons, hawks, eagles. Fortunately, these scenarios play out fairly swiftly. What concerned me was the extreme lack of water in the area. It's one thing to feed coyotes and quite another to allow an animal to die slowly of thirst. That seemed cruel. Passing by the refugee flock en route to the new dispensary location, Dusty and I chased the chickens around and around in a fowl attempt at rescuing the big hens but they proved elusive. On the way back we tried in vain once more to catch them but they emulated Br'er Rabbit, dashing swiftly into humanly inaccessible brambles. We never saw them again.

Dispirited

I was having one of those rare days where I felt downhearted to the point of mean. A day in which everything and everybody, including myself when I looked in the mirror, appeared ugly. A day where the slightest thing such as the damned tag on the back of my shirt irritated me. To be honest I'm not sure where these unpleasant feelings originated. Freud would have muttered something about my childhood, but my childhood had nothing at all to do with the way I felt that day. Perhaps deep down I felt frustrated about the dispensary or more specifically how each and every detail seemed to drag on for days and then weeks. These feelings were laced with a vague sense of guilt as I felt I should be doing something, anything to propel the business along. The sad fact was there wasn't much to do at the time. We were constantly waiting for *something*. Invariably this *something* was necessary before embarking on the next *something* we needed to accomplish. No water until we had electric to power the pump. The Internet and computer systems were also contingent on electric. However, when we finally had the power hooked up the internet company told us there was no service out where we were. 'Give us 45 days or so and we'll figure it out for you.' We had less than four weeks to obtain our operating license.

The clerk at the discount store commented on the *Yooper* shirt I was wearing, saying 'I was going to ask you where you got your shirt but you probably got it in the U.P.' I should have replied with something flowery such as 'Yes, it's very pleasant in that part of Michigan, are you from there?' She, or someone she knew obviously had to be from there or she wouldn't have recognized the slogan on the shirt. Instead, I just said 'yeah' and grabbed my bags from the counter.

The more I contemplated my foul mood, the more I began to think perhaps the dispensary had nothing to do whatsoever with my ill-temper. It being the first Saturday in June, weekenders occupied many normally vacant cabins and mobile homes up and down my street. In a fog of holiday-like merriment, the weekenders often drive up and down the road all day long raising clouds of dust in their wake. They were just having fun. There was no need for me to begrudge them. But I did anyway. This annoyance took me back to my youth, more specifically my college days at Kent State where we laughed at *Townies* who often voiced their displeasure with college kids defiling 'their town'. Now the shoe was squarely on the other foot, the roles having been reversed.

Maybe it wasn't the weekenders at all. It could quite possibly have been any one of the derelict idlers calling the neighborhood home. Whether traipsing around on foot or driving a beat automobile, these characters offer little to society. Most smoke meth, few, if any work, and each one of them appears more ignorant than the next. I'm no elitist snob, in fact I get along with virtually anyone, but it's difficult to even hold a conversation with one of these people for more than a few minutes. So it could have been that one of these people, driving aimlessly down the road set me off.

Or was it the squatters, friends or acquaintances of the aforementioned subculture, which had recently set up camp directly across the road from me in a dilapidated camping trailer lacking power or water. I wouldn't have minded it so much had they been campers and had in fact been camping but they were neither, merely a pack of idle squatters lacking the common sense or resources to contemplate their next move.

On the other hand, my vulgar disposition may have had something to do with the neighborhood cats producing horrible sounds all night. Though not as ghastly as the sounds emanating from the cats on the island of Nangan during my stint there, the eerily-humanlike sounds of mating certainly grates on a person's nerves after a while. Digging deeper for the truth, I don't believe the cacophony of odd utterances bothered me as much as the cats themselves. What began as a stray or two several years ago has evolved into a pride if such a word can be used to describe semi-feral felines. In my foul mood I angrily yet silently challenged the actions of charitable neighbors. By occasionally feeding and not actually taking in the stray band of marauders, these charitable people were merely prolonging a miserable situation. Lacking adequate shelter and warmth the mangy cats were continually cold, wet, and undernourished. What started out as an orange cat or two now took on every color imaginable. Grey, yellow, black, white, tiger-striped, Persian-ish, Siamese-ish, and of course more orange. In my present disposition I questioned whether it weren't more humane to round all the cats up and just get rid of them. It was only a matter of time before all these semi-feral cats procreated and there would be many more. Hell, even the coyotes will be outnumbered if this sort of thing goes on much longer. When I mentioned these mean-spirited notions to my wife she shuddered in horror. 'That's bad luck! Nobody would ever do that in Cambodia!' 'Well maybe they should, I countered. Aren't one or two healthy cats better than eighteen unhealthy ones?' My argument went nowhere. Like most people, my wife saw no benefit in exterminating a pack of stray cats even if it meant allowing them to suffer. My views were Hitleresque. Meanwhile, these charitable neighbors of mine are viewed as American versions of Mother Teresa; after all they're saving a pack of wild cats from extinction. Or are they? Could they, by their own good intentions, actually be torturing these ragamuffin cats? I suppose the answer is gray like one of the strays.

So what did I do to alleviate my distressed demeanor you ask? No, though I had inclinations, I didn't go out and start hunting down the stray cats. I took a deep breath and opened a beer. It was my way of dealing with things. It was a non-violent solution to an awful day. Gandhi would have been proud…At least about the non-violent approach. Let's just hope tomorrow is a better day as I don't have the money nor inclination to drink every day.

A Grow Facility Cometh...

In the midst of stringing electric to the property we stumbled across what we thought would be the answer to our growing needs, at least temporarily. On one of our many forty-minute trips over to Show Low to acquire odds and ends, I proposed we drop by the mobile home showroom to see if any used trailers had become available. It wasn't by any means a novel idea but we were becoming desperate for some solution to a grow facility. Noticing the used (and very dilapidated) doublewide in the lot, one that we had passed up on a previous visit, we inquired as to whether it was still available. It wasn't. But...it just so happened, another one was scheduled to become available that very day. As it wasn't yet on the lot we followed the owner of the business over to where it sat in a neighborhood on the other side of town. He warned us multiple times not to venture over by ourselves (meaning without him). He never explained why, but we assumed the mobile was a repo and he was afraid we'd be shot at by disgruntled exiles. To be honest, I'd never given much thought to the mobile home repo business. Cars sure, but mobile homes? I suppose it works along the lines of home foreclosure, when someone stops making their payments the bank or mobile home company in this case, steps in to secure their investment. Whereas site-built homes stay where they are, mobile homes are towed away. Like most (if not all) mobiles we'd looked at, a certain mildewy aroma emanated from the doorway as we hopped up to take a look around inside. The salesman eagerly declared that the 24' by 48' hulk was a 1980 Fuqua. Seeing this rang no bells he said it was similar to a (I'm making this up because I don't remember exactly what he said) Town and Country or an Old Towne Deluxe. As evidenced by the new subfloor, someone had begun remodeling. Cutting to the chase the salesman said it could be ours for only $9,200. By purchasing it that day we could have it delivered directly to our location and by doing so the owner could avoid having it brought over to his lot which meant he could sell it for much cheaper than it would go for once it was moved to his lot. By this time we understood the value of such an item and although to the uneducated eye the trailer appeared to be in shambles, it was a bargain. There were at least two other interested parties waiting in the wings. That may sound ridiculous but the market is rock solid for old smelly trailers. As my old friend Jim Fitzgerald would say, 'it was time to shit or get off the pot'.

Returning several hours later with a plastic shopping bag full of cash (the only way the deal could go down so said the trailer salesman) we sat around counting grubby bills until everyone was satisfied, even a small mongrel frolicking atop the salesman's desk. Plopping down the bag full of money was easy compared with getting the thing out to the location. For a fee of $4,200 a subcontractor named Jackie begrudgingly agreed (he wanted $4,800) to haul it out and set it up on blocks. There was a snag. His truck engine was being overhauled in Phoenix. He'd get it out to us as soon as he could. A week later he promised he'd 'be out on Monday'. I mentioned to Dusty that 'Monday' was Memorial Day and wondered if Jackie realized this. He didn't. Monday came and went with assurances that he'd be out the following Friday. After a largely civil disagreement, he agreed to come out on Thursday. By Friday the job had been completed and Dusty began stripping the place out. We had a grow facility. Was it optimal? Of course not, but it was a start. Pleased by the development we received word from the state that we'd have to pony up an additional $2,500 because we had changed locations. We explained that we had only changed locations because the county forced us out of town. It wasn't a voluntary change! Our protests fell on deaf ears.

PART IV

Final Push

Twisting Up Loose Ends

*T*hree weeks prior to what amounted to our deadline (the state inspection authorizing the license to operate) Heather and her son Ryan (AKA *Little Eddie*) arrived from Ohio. After selling her house and saying goodbye to family and friends Heather was all set for her new life as a dispensary owner. Or so she thought. Had we been allowed to open up in our intended location she would have been greeted with modernity and functionality. Instead, Heather found herself confronted by dysfunctional facilities and endless technological complications. Dusty and I, desensitized to a point of numbness, had been mired in obsolescence from the moment we had been banished to the hinterland months earlier. High-priced, hideous smelling, hauled-in well water. A woefully inadequate "high-speed" internet service. Substandard electrical amperage. Mud and cow patties. Zero shade. It served no useful purpose to bitch about it. We simply had to make the best of a lousy situation. The knowledge that we were still in the running was comforting, but deep down we understood our entry in the contest was far from blue ribbon material.

The emergence of Heather led to feelings of ambivalence on my part. On the one hand her boundless energy and ambition to get things done, no matter how long the hours or workload, was beneficial. On the other hand, this full-tilt drive of Heather's made me question whether the business would ever resemble anything approaching the concept of fun, something I saw as necessary in my participation. While working at the pawn shop I quickly realized having fun was essential. I'm not saying people didn't work hard, I'm simply saying the atmosphere at a pawn shop, as you might guess, is by nature gloomy, so to add to this gloominess with further gloominess would be, well, gloomy. I had agreed to participate in the business to A. help Dusty realize his dream, B. make money, and C. have fun along the way. The way I look at it, at my age, if a job isn't fun and relatively stress-free (at least from within), I'd just as soon be an idle pauper living in the woods – something I already profess to be.

Each day of mindless toil, *polishing the turd as it were*, brought us one step nearer to completion. The dispensary, no matter how hard we tried, was never going to be anything more than functional. The word *chic* would never be used to describe the place. It is impossible to produce gems from a lump of coal. There was only so much we could do with an venerable doublewide and a leased construction trailer. A few coats of paint inside and out. A little (we only had enough material for half the mobile) metal skirting around the bottom. A new wood floor in the grow facility. Spreading wood chips over the muddy, cow-chippy field that served as the parking lot. The touch-ups and buffing seemed to go on interminably until one day it all stopped. There was no more to do. Rather, it was as good as it would ever get.

In order to qualify for the state inspection we had first to obtain a final inspection from the county allowing us to occupy the facility. Accustomed to residential building codes, Dusty and I were unaware of everything that was required of us and therefore failed the inspection the first time around. We had erroneously believed that the inspector would come out and examine whether we had properly installed the sewer and electrical lines. As for the illuminated and battery-backed up exit signs and fire escape maps, we hadn't a clue. The inclusion of a handicap accessible ramp leading into the front dispensary was the most daunting item on the inspector's list. This was something I had feared and expected all along as I had once, many years earlier, carried out ADA compliance inspections for a private company at state parks throughout the state. Upon mentioning the glaring oversight I was told repeatedly by Bob and Heather, who assured they were handling the issue, that it would be wise to wait and see whether anyone noticed. Low and behold the inspector noticed and it cost $1600 to install the ramp, which by the way was still less costly than renting a steel one for $250 a month with a one-year contract. Making a phone call to Monty, our cow-owning/insurance agent neighbor to the west, we were able to find a carpenter to come out on short notice to assemble the ramp. Just as we were wondering whether the contractor would even show, he arrived with a crew of ten or twelve. Three hours later the ramp was complete. With the ramp out of the way we easily crossed the other minor deficiencies off the list and were able to obtain the permit of occupancy. The only obstacle remaining was the state inspection.

The original state inspection was slated for July 23rd. I wasn't sure whether to treat the state-selected date, which just so happened to coincide with the date of my birth, as a portent of good fortune or a harbinger of doom. In the end it didn't much matter as the inspection was moved back a day to July 24th. In retrospect I should have welcomed the intrusion upon my birthday as we spent over 12 hours on the 23rd ironing out various problems with the surveillance system. The problems we were experiencing stemmed not from the system itself but from a serious lack of internet bandwidth. Due to the remoteness of the location our lifeline to the World Wide Web remained sketchy at best. Though we were able to access a cable service, the strength of the signal, taxed as it were by the extent it was required to travel to reach us, teetered on the brink of inoperability. Whereas download speeds hovered near adequate ranges, upload speeds – essential for viewing the cameras online – were virtually nonexistent. After making several calls to the surveillance system manufacturer, I resigned myself to the fact that there was really nothing more I could do. There was nothing wrong with the system and therefore no one to blame. When the state came to inspect the system, we'd have to cross our fingers and hope the page displaying the images would hold before disappearing into that dreaded *This page can't be displayed* or *You're not connected to a network* mode. That, or pray an electrical storm covered up our technological shortcomings.

The three-member state inspection team arrived sometime after eleven o'clock. Arriving in two vehicles the trio, two men and a woman, gazed at their surroundings as if in a dream. 'You guys weren't kidding when you said you were out in the middle of nowhere', exclaimed the female inspector. In the pretense of state efficiency (an oxymoron perhaps), the inspectors split their team, sending the two male inspectors, one of them in training, with Dusty and I to demonstrate the security and surveillance systems while the female inspector, who was nominally in charge, met with Heather and Bob to go over the policies and procedures. I could feel the tension mounting as I stepped over to the computer to demonstrate the monitoring system. Easing the mood with small-talk banter, I attempted to deflect glances from the screen until I was able to bring up the camera images. Temporarily getting the page to stick without dissolving I proudly showed the inspector the various storefront views. Aside from a camera angle he requested to be tweaked (Dusty quickly climbing a ladder to do so); the inspector gave the impression he was pleased with both the screen display and coverage offered by the cameras. After a nervous second or two waiting for a color photo to spit out from the printer (there had been issues with that as well), I crossed my fingers and prayed that I could pull up images from the second set of cameras located in the back grow-house. As I said, the system worked flawlessly (aside from occasional printing problems), it was the internet that we relied on to display the images that was insufficient. I caught a glimpse of Dusty across the counter as he stood there trying not to act nervous, all the while knowing the slightest misstep could derail the entire inspection. After ten or so covert clicks of the mouse I was finally able to raise the screen and show the inspector the range of images depicted across it. I knew it was inevitable that the screen would eventually go blank, I just didn't know when. Nervously awaiting the command to print a still image from the back cameras, I was relieved when the inspector announced it was time to take a tour of the grow facility and camera locations. Our luck had held, we had squeaked by. Albeit barely.

The remainder of the inspection went off without a hitch with only three minor deficiencies standing in the way of opening the doors. The first was a simple document stating that we hadn't done any business in 2012. Why this was deemed necessary was beyond my comprehension as it was clear we hadn't been open for business in 2012 as we were still yet to open for business and here it was July, 2013. The second concern centered around the need of an audible warning when a surveillance camera went down. Had I known it was as simple as it proved to be I would have remedied the problem while the inspectors stood in front of the monitor. As it was, I quickly fixed the problem the following morning by clicking a few boxes in the DVR's menu.

The final deficiency required a signature by the sheriff's office on a document stating that they were informed by us that they would be called in the case of emergency. The next morning we drove down to the main sheriff's office in Holbrook to acquire the signature. Met at the window by a brusque, no-nonsense female, we explained our situation. Her facial expression, painfully serious if not grim, never once wavered during the exchange. As we stood there listening to the gears click in her head I imagined her possessing an uncanny aptitude for poker. Informing us she was personally unauthorized to sign the paper, which again was nothing more than a sentence or two explaining we would add the department's number to our alarm system, the gloomy woman begrudgingly left the window to seek assistance. Returning, she said she had placed the document on the sheriff's desk for signature. That was the best she could do for us. 'How long will it take for him to sign it, I asked? Shrugging her rigid frame, she replied with a catty snuffle: 'I haven't the faintest idea.' Seeing there was nothing more to say we jumped back in Heather's car and drove the forty odd miles back to the dispensary. Not about to let such a triflingly small detail hold us back we printed out another copy of the document and made haste for the Navajo County Sheriff's Department substation in Overgaard. Knowing that the substation is a non-public office, I had doubts as to whether anyone would even answer the buzzer. Standing near the door in an attempt to discern activity from within, it appeared we were out of luck as no one came to answer. Then, just as we turned to leave a shadow, then an arm, then a uniformed figure emerged from the doorway. Though the officer, who I took for a reserve member of the department, was heads and tails more cheery than the woman at the Holbrook office, he too said he was unauthorized to sign the document. Picking up on our frustration (we had already told him we had driven to Holbrook and back) he agreed to make a phone call to his commanding officer. Five minutes later he emerged with the document, signed by non-other than himself. Apparently the commanding officer had no qualms whatsoever. Better yet, why would he? It was just a silly piece of paper stating that we would call the police if so required.

Deficiencies cleared up, we were given the go ahead from the state to open our doors.

~

Overgaard Compassion Care officially opened its doors to the cardholding public on Thursday, August 1, 2013. There were no balloons or noisemakers. Nor were there any eye-popping pyrotechnic displays or hot dogs smeared with brown mustard. Having pushed so hard to finish up by the deadline, we hadn't even had a chance to acquire a scale. Undeterred, we waited impatiently for customers to arrive. Problem was, preparations were not made in the area of advertising thus there was little hope of anyone paying the storefront a visit. A banner announcing that we were open for business had been hung and in a typical, citified setting, this might have sufficed. But when you're located out in the middle of nowhere, like we were, that banner screwed to the side of the building was like a buoy placed out in open water – thoughtful, but not very practical.

A total of six people entered the shop that day, three of which bought varying amounts of medicinal-grade marijuana. As for the other three: One guy stopped by to have a look around. Another, wearing kneepads, said he had been working on the cell tower next door and was curious. Grinning, the man asked: 'How to I buy some?' The sixth of the six prospective shoppers was a salesman who dropped by to offer glimpses of a new cannabis product line. With arms as big as an average man's legs, the man was a dead ringer for John Coffey in *The Green Mile*. You normally envision a man that large driving a proportionately-sized vehicle, so you can imagine my astonishment when he arrived in a Mini Cooper.

Altercation at the Compactor

*I*t had become fairly commonplace for people to display displeasure, even hostility toward us for opening up a medical marijuana dispensary in Heber-Overgaard. On the other hand, it was virtually unheard of for anyone bearing a pro-marijuana stance to display passionate antagonism toward us for doing so. This novel form of vehemence was chiefly brought about because the opening of a dispensary in the area signaled financial ruin as cultivators lost their grow rights. Awareness of this new set of adversaries confronted our consciousness one morning as Dusty and I dropped off a load of malodorous rubbish at the community trash compactor – a machine attached to the end of a loading dock designed to smash up refuse before being sent off to a landfill. In the process of shedding several bags of trash a guy walked beside Dusty, making cheery comments surrounding the carpentry tools in the back of his truck. He merrily mentioned that he too was in the trades. In the midst of this running commentary the guy happened to notice the hood of a large grow light nestled up near the cab which gave rise to yet another remark: 'Oh, you're a fellow grower!' Seizing the opportunity to market the dispensary Dusty explained that we had state-regulated dispensary rights in the area and would soon be opening up the storefront. What should have been heartwarming news was taken as anything but by the man who soon went into an excitable and invective tirade on the subject of dispensaries. This fit of sorts was made all the worse when Dusty informed him we'd be doing our best to open by the 24th of July. Mention of the date brought blood to the man's face as he begged us to open up after the 1st of August so that he could renew his cultivator's permit for another year. We explained that we had no control over the date the state had specified to conduct their inspection. While the man told us he didn't dislike us personally, something he uttered far too many times to be believable, he admonished that he along with "300 other people were pissed off as hell" that the dispensary was opening at all as it was going to put them all out of business or at least bar them from growing marijuana in their homes. Dusty told the guy he sympathized with him as we (and everyone else) knew it would come to that eventually. This was of course the whole point of the dispensary system: To bring home grows to a halt. After repeating himself thirty times pertaining to how 'pissed off he was' and 'how he didn't blame us personally...But', the man, who was perhaps our age – in his mid to late forties – said he'd have to pick up and move farther out of town to escape the 25-mile radius 'no-grow' shadow cast by our dispensary. 'I've moved before and I guess I'll have to do it again.' Knowing there was nothing I could say to assuage the man's ill temper, I didn't say anything. It was obvious that aside from being more than a little nutty the guy was on the verge of meltdown. Feeling there was no need for any violence at the trash compactor; Dusty did his best to placate the man by soothing him with as much sympathy as one can when parked near wafting aromas of spoiled food and decomposing cardboard.

The man declared (at least eight times) that 'he didn't grow the marijuana to sell or trade', insisting that he only grew what he needed in order to satisfy his condition. As to what that condition was I couldn't readily ascertain, perhaps chronic pain as this seems to be the predominant factor in obtaining a medical marijuana card in the state of Arizona. We said we understood and sympathized, even going so far as to offer condolences. What more could we say? What I didn't comment on were the faulty lines of reasoning behind his statement that he would have to 'move' as if he'd been a homesteader with marijuana growing rights for the past half century. The medical marijuana laws had passed in November of 2010 but hadn't gone into effect in the form of cards enabling a person to cultivate until months later. In other words the man could only have been legally growing his own supply for perhaps two years at most. The way he made it sound, his pappy and his grand pappy before him had been sharecropping the land for years. When, in the midst of one of his rants he let slip that he lived 15 miles out of town I immediately pegged him as a stalwart resident of Chevelon Retreat, a grid-eschewing populous renown for growing marijuana – both legally and illegally. I was wrong on that account but wouldn't realize it until several weeks later.

Just as I thought the man, who had been planted on the passenger side of the truck bellowing into my ear for some time by now, was going to leave (he had gotten back into his car), he came racing back out for another round of ranting and raving, tiny drops of spittle spewing from the corners of his incensed orifice. This time around the histrionics had mainly to do with the state police and their campaign to crack down on card-holding medical marijuana patients. Displaying his medical marijuana card once more (this made three times), he went on to dispel truths, half-truths, and rumors regarding the current stance of the state police (Department of Public Safety, better known as DPS) pertaining to smoking marijuana and driving. I'd long known there were problems with the way the police in Arizona and many other states determine whether or not a person is under the influence. With the scrutiny of a blood test a person could be rendered under the influence of marijuana even if they hadn't smoked or ingested any cannabis products for days, even weeks, as a metabolite known as Carboxy-THC remains enmeshed in the body's fatty tissue for extended periods of time. Thus, the more fat on your frame the longer THC will remain in your system. Some states have wisely opted for innovative blood tests which can fairly accurately determine whether a person was high at the time of being pulled over or merely had marijuana in their bloodstream. There is of course a huge difference between toking up two minutes ago and toking up two weeks ago. As of today law enforcement in Arizona makes no distinction between the two. Making his position on all things cannabis known both to us and anyone else who was of a mind to listen, the man mercifully climbed into his car and left us in peace.

~

Based on what I have just said, you can imagine my great surprise, when one morning soon after opening, who should appear but the irate ear-bender from the compactor. I immediately recognized him as soon as I saw him driving into the parking lot. Cringing, I awaited the onslaught I knew was coming – how we'd wronged him and his fellow home-growing brethren. Pulling in behind the building, I assume so no one saw him pull in, he slowly made his way around to the storefront. Catching a glimpse of our visitor, Dusty made haste in the other direction by seeking refuge in the grow facility. Fearing the worst, I calmed myself for what I perceived to be yet another battering. The encounter, though somewhat starchy at the onset, softened considerably as I accompanied the man outside after a short tour of the facility. Once outside we delved into what can only be described as an agreeable conversation. There was no ranting or raving. Before me stood a civilized individual with articulate thoughts. He spoke of growing up in Santa Cruz, California and having been raised in and around marijuana. So much so, that he considered from a very young age that the substance was legal as everyone around him was so casually involved with it. We spoke of the many benefits and challenges presented by growing marijuana in a climate such as this – warm summers, cold winters, the effects of altitude and so on.

Several minutes into our conversation I expressed the view that based on our earlier encounter I had him pegged for a class-A lunatic. I wasn't at all sure how he might take this bold depiction or why I felt the nagging need to convey this observation at that particular moment. Standing across from one another on the freshly constructed, state-mandated thirty-foot wheelchair ramp, a structure which could easily have doubled for a bridge over a crocodile-infested moat, I steadied myself for the man's emotive reply to my risqué declaration. Would he reply with another explosive, rage-filled tirade or sheepish laughter? Fortunately it was the latter. Explaining in broad detail his feelings and frame of mind that particular morning at the compactor, the Santa Cruz native offered a sly grin, acknowledging he must have appeared a bit crazy at the time. 'A *bit*,' I joked. What do you know; the guy I had pegged for a lunatic wasn't half bad.

The Mutie Chart

*I*t is not my intention here to debauch the medical marijuana industry. I have nothing to gain by doing so. What I'm about to discuss is based solely on my own perceptions and observations. I am neither a physician nor a scientist. Nor am I someone claiming to possess lay expertise (trust me, these people are out there) in either of the two fields. I'm merely an attentive individual who believes in honest, unbiased reasoning. Having laid down my disclaimer, let's discuss some of the idiosyncrasies I find within the "medical" scope of medical marijuana. While there appears to be supportive evidence suggesting that medical marijuana treats and soothes a wide variety of various conditions the debate rages on as to whether medical marijuana actually cures any of them. As a pragmatist, I often find myself crouching in an extremely conservative position when it comes to cure-alls of any kind. Images of snake-oil salesmen come to mind. As a free-thinking individual, I believe there should be no boundary, certainly no interferential governmental boundary, left unbreached when it comes to curing illness. If cannabis or any other substance, natural or unnatural, eases someone's pain or improves their quality of life, I believe it should be made readily available. Why should anyone have to suffer unnecessarily?

I can't begin to tell you how many times I've squirmed in my seat at a restaurant listening to self-important know-it-alls enthusiastically describe the processes by which marijuana has 'cured' people of this or that illness. Not only did it ease someone's pain but actually 'cured' it. 'I swear this woman had a cancerous area right here on her right forearm. After several treatments with cannabis-based products (lotions and potions) the cancer completely cleared out. It was unbelievable!' I concur. It was unbelievable.

Earlier in the book I listed some of the conditions treated by cannabis and cannabis-related products. Aids, cancer, glaucoma, hepatitis, epilepsy, migraine headaches, spasms, sleep disorders, chronic pain; the list goes on and on. The way I see it, treating and curing are two very different concepts. If cannabis had the capacity to 'cure', not only treat, but "cure", diseases such as AIDS and cancer there is no way in the world that any government could (or should) prevent someone from getting their hands on it through one means or another, legally or otherwise. If I was inflicted with AIDS and was told there was a cure out there, I'd find a way to get my hands on it even if it meant breaking laws. What do you have to lose? What sort of fair and just system precludes people from a healthy existence? In a nut shell, this is the basis for the debate on medical marijuana. Is the system abused? Of course it is. Are there people out there recreating in the name of medicating? Of course there are. Name me a social system that isn't abused. Welfare?

Fibromyalgia is another hotly contested condition treated by medical marijuana. Fibromyalgia, sometimes referred to as FM or FMS, is a mysterious condition characterized by chronic pain found throughout the body. I say mysterious because no one seems to know for certain what exactly causes the condition. According to scientists and physicians the source of fibromyalgia can be traced to genetic, neurobiological, psychological, and environmental factors. With factors as diverse as these it is obviously difficult to get a firm grasp on the condition. In addition to widespread chronic pain fibromyalgia sufferers may also encounter symptoms of fatigue, joint stiffness and soreness, sleep disturbance, depression, anxiety, muscle numbness and tingling, bowel and bladder abnormality, and even cognitive dysfunction. Fibromyalgia, believed to affect 2-4% of the population, affects each person differently and seems to afflict women disproportionately (as much as 9:1).

Not long ago we were approached by a man claiming to have solved the riddle. Not only had he found a strain that eased the symptoms of fibromyalgia, but more significantly, had cured it. In two weeks' time no less! Was I skeptical? Of course I was. This man wasn't a scientist or physician, he was a businessman. He rattled off impressive numbers and statistics while describing lavish plans to corner the market. Let's assume, just for the sake of argument, that there were 20,000 fibromyalgia patients in Arizona. From a business standpoint ridding all these people of fibromyalgia was an enormous coup. In financial terms it would certainly mean millions to whoever was able to somehow corner the market. As I stood there listening, I wondered why this forward-thinking businessman hadn't considered the ramifications, or lack thereof in this instance, for repeat business. If every would-be fibromyalgia patient were cured there would be no need for further treatment, or consequently, sales. It was a one and done deal. Unless someone suffered a relapse, but if that occurred, then we can't assume they were ever actually 'cured'.

Fortunately, I have a simple solution for making heads and tails of each, and well, almost every condition known to man that is either *treated* or *cured* by marijuana-based products. My brainchild, known as the Mutie Chart (named after my colorfully copyrighted mutant surf-punker cartoon character), allows me to accurately determine which strain or edible concoction will be most effective for any given scenario. Lower back pain you say? Let's see, it looks as if White Widow will work wonders on that. Shingles? Eat half this chocolate chip cookie followed by a vapor hit or two of Banana Kush. Gout? According to the Mutie Chart here it looks as if Green Crack should do. In need of an attitude adjustment? Mr. Nice Guy can take care of that. Amnesia? Well sir, it doesn't seem as though the Mutie Chart has yet accounted for that condition. So sorry about that, but hold the phone, I'll see what I can do. One moment please while I consult with someone in back. Ehem, sir, I have it on good authority that Crystal Diesel neatly fits the bill for amnesia. However, if you are unable to remember this recommendation then I presume any old strain ought to suffice.

In all seriousness, if it works it works.

Same, Same, But Different

Anyone who has traveled throughout Southeast Asia is undoubtedly familiar with the phrase *Same, Same, but Different*. It adorns t-shirts and can be often heard in conversations with locals, especially in market settings. At its core the phrase makes absolutely no sense. How can any one thing, or concept for that matter, be identical yet different? In locations such as Siem Reap, Cambodia and Chiang Mai, Thailand the phrase frequently implies or describes items of a similar nature. For instance, a knock-off Rolex in the Old Market may be peddled as *same, same, but different*. Used in this context the phrase almost makes sense. Almost. The phrase may also be employed to describe men portraying themselves as women, a cultural set known as Ladyboys. Entirely convincing at times, these transsexual males frequently catch inebriated tourists off guard. Expecting one thing, a drunken male tourist suddenly receives the shock of his life when he learns the beautiful woman he's been dancing with all night is actually a man. Embarrassed, he implores a befriended local to clear things up. Shrugging his shoulders the befriended local sighs before replying *same, same, but different*.

By now you're probably wondering where all this is headed and better yet, how it can possibly tie into a book about marijuana. An observant people-watcher, very early on I began taking stock of the various people purchasing medical marijuana. In doing so I couldn't seem to shake an uncanny feeling of familiarity, that I'd somehow met some of these people somewhere before. Perhaps not *them* personally, but someone similar to *them*. Someone *same, same, but different*. But where? Then it dawned on me. Many of the dispensary customers appeared similar to the people I had dealt with on a daily basis down at the pawn shop. They also were similar to people I often encountered at a good friend's tattoo shop. I am in no way insinuating this was a bad thing – most are great to converse with – it was just eerie was all. Not normally one to pigeon-hole people as one thing or another, I found myself entranced by these peculiar ponderings. Was it possible that the dispensary clientele were in fact *same, same, but different*? This is not to say that anyone traveled exclusively in these well-ordered circles; that would be asking a lot, perhaps even too much. On the other hand, it would not at all be a great leap of faith to propose correlations exist.

These quirky musings led me to additional quirky musings. As I stood there behind the counter acting as *budtender*, a term, by the way, I happen to loathe, I considered the profound influence the medical marijuana era is having on the manner in which 'medicine' is distributed. Standing behind a counter filled with jars containing a myriad of different strains of marijuana, I had the occasion to smile at the stark contrast drawn between medical marijuana dispensaries and medicinal 'peddlers' of yore. I cheekily use the word yore but we all know many of these 'peddlers still exist and always will. Just for fun let's tag along with *Roger* as he shops for his medicine. As a longtime roofer, Roger experiences what he refers to as chronic back pain.

Scenario One:

After visiting an ATM Roger heads for an apartment complex several miles distant. It's ten am on a Tuesday morning. Calling ahead, Roger is given the green light to approach the apartment. Making sure his car is locked, Roger looks cautiously around wondering if he's being watched. Roger's rap on the door is scrutinized by a wary eye through a peephole. Locks are soon manipulated and Roger steps out of the sunlight into the relative darkness of the apartment. With the curtains and blinds drawn and a hint of mustiness filling the air, it takes several moments for Roger's eyes to adjust to the obscurity of the cave-like atmosphere. An ever-present drone emanates from a television set sitting atop a makeshift stand. The set rarely powers down. Scanning the room Roger notices remnants of the past in the form of crusty plates, overflowing ashtrays, and empty potato chip bags. It is apparent Roger's host has recently awakened. Then, he may look similarly disheveled at four in the afternoon. The dealer's level of hygiene is of no importance to the visitor, who'll soon be of a mind to overlook such trivialities. Omnipresent and duty-bound, the dealer has no life of his own. Partaking with every new patron, the dealer's day progresses at the unhurried pace of the pipe load. As the customer, typically a friend, or friend of a friend, which is the case with Roger, plops down on the couch, the ritual begins. The host, reaching down between his legs, swings open a small cabinet door on his side of the coffee table. Adeptly producing a tray containing his latest acquisition, he offers a whiff. Unlike today's modern houses of pot the selection at the host's establishment is rather narrow. One takes

211

what one can get. Opening up an adjacent cabinet door the dealer produces a glass bong. Depending on the time of day and hygienic habits of the dealer, the vessel may or may not be clean. Samples are loaded and passed around. Comments are made on the product's texture, taste, and smell. Or lack thereof. Following a brief, one-sided discussion as to the price the host stuffs a baggie and tosses it across the coffee table to Roger, who robotically places it in his hip pocket. Formalities out of the way, both Roger and his host gaze up at the images being emitted from the idiot box. Bob Barker is receiving a peck on the cheek from a showcase showdown winner. As Roger exits the apartment the world takes on a surreal quality. A slight bout of paranoia grips him as he backs out his car and pulls out of the complex. Unbeknownst to Roger, another guest is at that very moment making his way into the parking lot from the far side of the complex. As each customer enters, the play commences anew. The sample tray appears and the dance begins.

Scenario Two:

Though Roger's been seeking solace for his discomfort through marijuana for years, this is his first visit to a state-regulated medical marijuana dispensary. Pulling into the parking lot Roger notices no discernible difference between the medical marijuana dispensary he is about to enter and the cash checking establishment he visited earlier that morning. Both are outwardly clean and secure. Like the check cashing joint, cameras record Roger's every move. After spending several minutes in a waiting area, Roger produces his state-issued medical marijuana card and is casually ushered into a 'selection room' where a friendly female employee adorned with facial jewelry stands waiting patiently behind a glass counter. Roger's eyes take it all in. One thing's for sure, he's not at the check cashing store. With so many options assaulting Roger's mind he allows the dispensary agent behind the counter to assist him in making a choice. The decision comes down to Northern Lights, Lemon Haze, and B52. It's a tough choice but Roger selects the Lemon Haze. He's not really sure why, perhaps he just wanted to get the hell out of there. The Haze is placed into a small shopping bag. After paying at the cash register, Roger walks back out to his parked car and drives home. Soberly. Everything had been perfectly legal.

Postscript

It's far too early to determine how successful the enterprise will turn out. A medical marijuana dispensary, like any business, requires time to nurture. Time, literally, to take root. I'd love to exclaim 'the sky's the limit' but the realist in me simply won't allow it. Each and every dispensary is limited by basic economic principles such as supply and demand. These factors are ultimately determined by price and quality. Affluence in medical marijuana all comes down to *the grow*. Without frequent and bountiful harvests a dispensary is hamstrung and left for dead. True, it's possible to buy product from other dispensaries and sell it at a modest profit, but the only way to make *a lot* of money doing so is to sell like crazy a la Wal-Mart. Problem is, a dispensary has only so many customers and dispensaries aren't buying their product from China. In other words, unless you're Wal-Mart, growing your own product line is absolutely essential to survival.

A friend recently asked: 'If you had it do all over again, would you?' That's a difficult question. One that I've asked myself many times. Can I offer a noncommittal *maybe*? There was certainly an educational component to the venture, though some of my newly acquired knowledge was grotesquely unsolicited. This might seem odd coming from a former civics teacher but my leeriness toward bureaucratic procedure was not assuaged in the least during the lengthy ordeal. While I wouldn't swap political systems with any other country in the world, this doesn't mean that there aren't shortcomings inherent to our own. Plenty of them. Politics at any level are precariously atilt. In rural settings where diversity of opinion tends to be at a minimum, political views often lose range and scope. You can hardly blame local politicians for refusing to stick their necks out over an unpopular issue. Based on pro-medical marijuana turnout at the county meetings I'd hazard to guess elected officials aren't overly concerned with losing votes.

Pioneers in any field, and pioneers in medical marijuana we certainly were, are bound to face challenge and adversity. The passage of laws doesn't necessarily equate to societal acceptance. Societal acceptance, like the growth of a business, requires time. Were people of color treated with due respect immediately following civil rights legislation? Were women treated as equals after given the right to vote? No and no. Passing a law sanctioning medical marijuana by no means equates to societal acceptance. A stepping stone toward legalization? Yes. Societal acceptance? No. Some stances will soften with each new generation. Some attitudes toward marijuana, medical or otherwise, will never change. It goes without saying that when dealing with a product, which for so many years has been out and out illegal, there is bound to be a fair degree of social stigma. You never knew what reaction might be evoked from someone when you told them what type of business you were starting up. Whether down at the water or electric company or down at the local hardware store, someone invariably asked what kind of business we were working on. Some took it in stride and laughed. Others did not. You may recall that the local newspaper attended our community meeting. When we contacted them regarding advertising they balked, worried that ads for marijuana might cause their customer base to melt away. In all honesty, some customers probably would have pulled out. The newspaper graciously offered to run a story but didn't offer to come out and actually conduct an interview and write one up. The last I heard Bob was working on writing one up. What the hell do I know about such things – after all, I'm only a former newspaper editor. So it goes, I suppose.

I'm often asked for my personal take on medical marijuana. More specifically, what I think about the concept of medical marijuana and its place in society. I often reply: If it helps someone they should have access to it. Invariably someone will snicker and say something like: 'Yeah but that can be said about recreational use as well couldn't it?' My stock reply: If it helps someone they should have access to it. If it were up to me, and it's obviously not, marijuana would be legal, regulated similarly to alcohol, with age limits and industry standards. There would be no need to define it as medicinal or recreational. Call it what it is: Using marijuana. Prison overpopulation would be eased. Cartels softened with the understanding that they would never become obsolete until drugs such as heroin and cocaine were legalized. Would marijuana usage witness an upswing? Possibly. But by how much and for how long? Alcohol is legal but that doesn't mean society, the city of Holbrook, Arizona excluded, collectively stumbles through life in a stupor.

In light of recent policy decisions made by the federal government to maintain a hands-off approach to

Colorado and Washington's legalization of recreational marijuana, many other states are currently scrambling to follow suit by gathering the required signatures to place the measure on future ballots. A grassroots organization calling itself 'Safer Arizona' is currently attempting to gather the 259,213 signatures required to bring the issue to a November, 2014 vote here in Arizona. Even Arizona Senator John McCain, historically a staunch advocate to marijuana, has recently softened his stance by admitting perhaps it is time to legalize. In a town hall meeting in Arizona McCain stated: 'Maybe we should legalize. We're certainly moving that way as far as marijuana is concerned. I respect the will of the people'

I'm often asked is whether or not marijuana, from a medical standpoint, actually benefits people. I'm not a doctor and I don't suffer from a chronic condition so I'm not in the best position to offer judgment. But from what I've witnessed and from what I've read, marijuana does appear to relieve symptoms of certain conditions. As I mentioned earlier in the book, I'm guardedly skeptical as to marijuana 'curing' conditions. I'm not saying it hasn't happened, I just haven't witnessed it personally. Consequently I remain unconvinced. Relief? Certainly. Cure? I'm not sure. Put it this way, I believe there is a strong possibility that extraterrestrial life exists. The universe is simply too vast for me to state without a shadow of a doubt that we are 'it'. Like claims of marijuana curing people of their illnesses, I have yet to have had a close encounter with an alien.

Despite the many benefits offered by marijuana, there is one thing it is not; a PED (performance enhancing drug). Not in my book anyway. Marijuana use does not equate to increased performance reviews at work. Nor does it assist in athletic training or higher test scores. While marijuana may well help an artist 'find her groove' or a songwriter 'lay out the lyrics' on his next big hit single, I doubt very much that it is beneficial to the neurosurgeon or the school bus driver.

~

No matter what happens, whether the dispensary rakes in millions or goes belly up, Dusty's dream was realized. That's the important thing. My work here done, it's time to get back to doing what I enjoy most…Traveling the world.

Overgaard, Arizona
September, 2013

Books by the Author

Man On The Scene series...

Man On The Scene	Malfeasance in Motion	
Slippery Escarpment	Another One More	
Best Of	Quixotic	Kaliu

Other works...

Vignettes from the Village

Scattered Thoughts

An Arizona 'Royal'... *The Life and Times of King S. Woolsey*

Opinions Are Like Anthills

Black Hills Invasion... *An Outsider's take on the Sturgis Rally*

Arun

Pawndemonium

About the Author

Jeff Quinn resides in a shack atop an escarpment in Eastern Arizona known as the Mogollon Rim. Always up for an adventure, Quinn enjoys traveling the world in search of history, culture, and colorful characters.

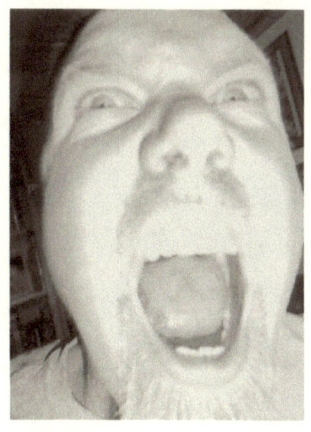

The author can be contacted through his website at
manonthescene.org

www.ingramcontent.com/pod-product-compliance
Lightning Source LLC
Chambersburg PA
CBHW050441290526
45786CB00006B/2111